Solutions for Weight Loss with Recipes of Mediterranean Diet

Tips for creating your own Menus

Sasha Merianelli

Table of Contents

Garlic Shrimp Fettuccine

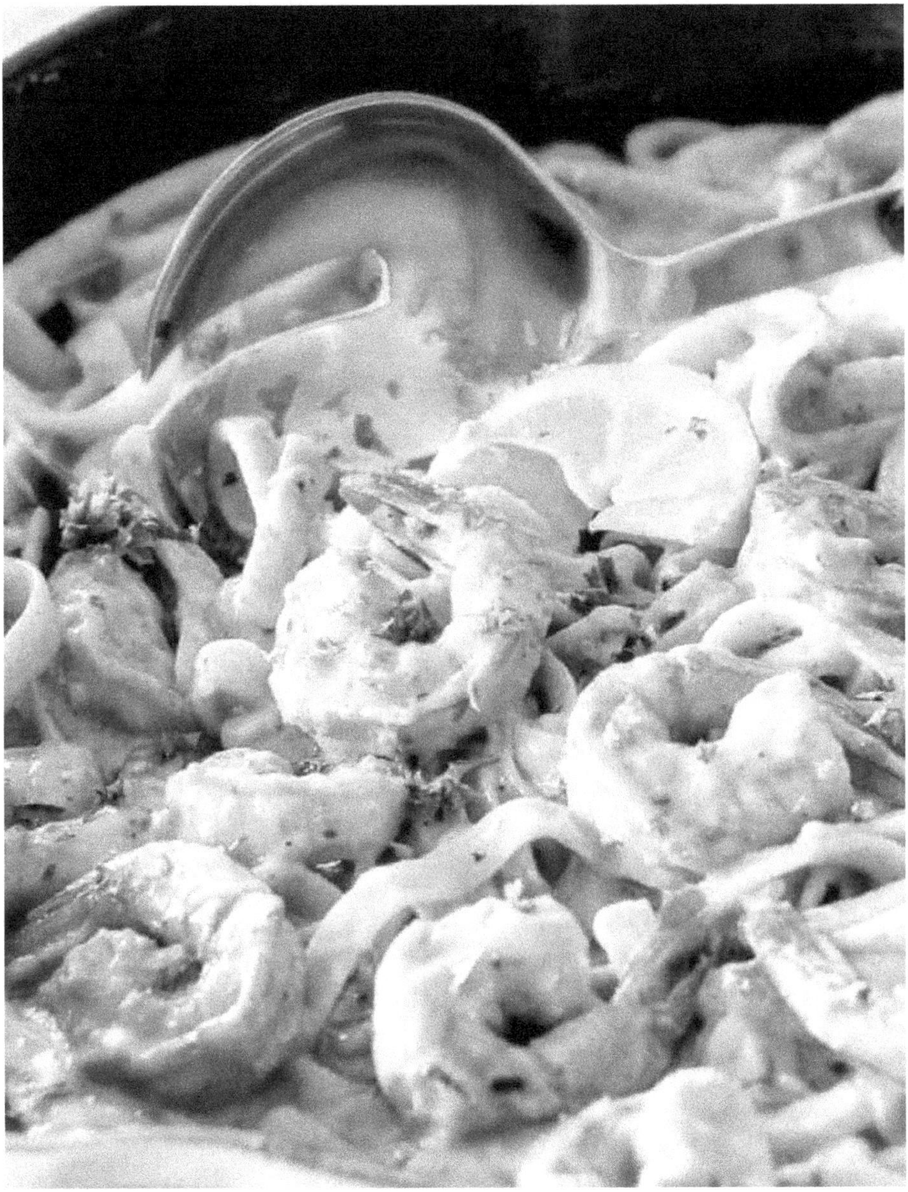

Prep time:

10 minutes | Cook time: 15 minutes | Serves 4 to 6

Ingredients

8 ounces (227 g) fettuccine pasta

¼ cup extra-virgin olive oil

3 tablespoons garlic, minced

1 pound (454 g) large shrimp, peeled and deveined

⅓ cup lemon juice

1 tablespoon lemon zest

½ teaspoon salt

½ teaspoon freshly ground black pepper

Direction

1. Bring a large pot of salted water to a boil. Add the fettuccine and cook for 8 minutes. Reserve ½ cup of the cooking liquid and drain the pasta.
2. In a large saucepan over medium heat, heat the olive oil. Add the garlic and sauté for 1 minute.
3. Add the shrimp to the saucepan and cook each side for 3 minutes. Remove the shrimp from the pan and set aside.
4. Add the remaining Ingredients to the saucepan. Stir in the cooking liquid. Add the pasta and toss together to evenly coat the pasta.
5. Transfer the pasta to a serving dish and serve topped with the cooked shrimp.

Per Serving

Calories: 615 | fat: 17.0g | protein: 33.0g | carbs: 89.0g | fiber: 4.0g | sodium: 407mg

Pesto Pasta

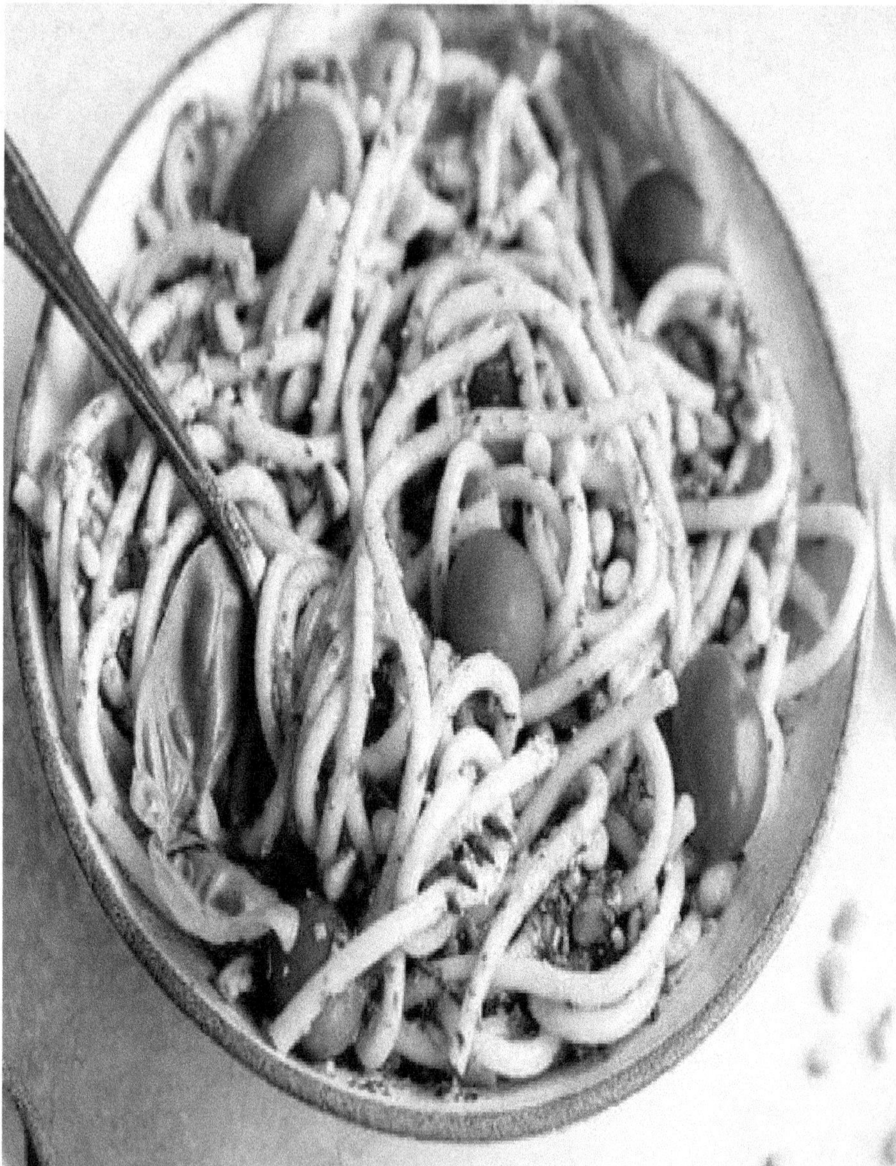

Prep time:

10 minutes | Cook time: 8 minutes | Serves 4 to 6

Ingredients

1 pound (454 g) spaghetti

4 cups fresh basil leaves, stems removed

3 cloves garlic

1 teaspoon salt

½ teaspoon freshly ground black pepper

½ cup toasted pine nuts

¼ cup lemon juice

½ cup grated Parmesan cheese

1 cup extra-virgin olive oil

Direction

1. Bring a large pot of salted water to a boil. Add the spaghetti to the pot and cook for 8 minutes.
2. In a food processor, place the remaining Ingredients, except for the olive oil, and pulse.
3. While the processor is running, slowly drizzle the olive oil through the top opening. Process until all the olive oil has been added.
4. Reserve ½ cup of the cooking liquid. Drain the pasta and put it into a large bowl. Add the pesto and cooking liquid to the bowl of pasta and toss everything together.
5. Serve immediately.

Per Serving

Calories: 1067 | fat: 72.0g | protein: 23.0g | carbs: 91.0g | fiber: 6.0g | sodium: 817mg

Spaghetti with Pine Nuts and Cheese

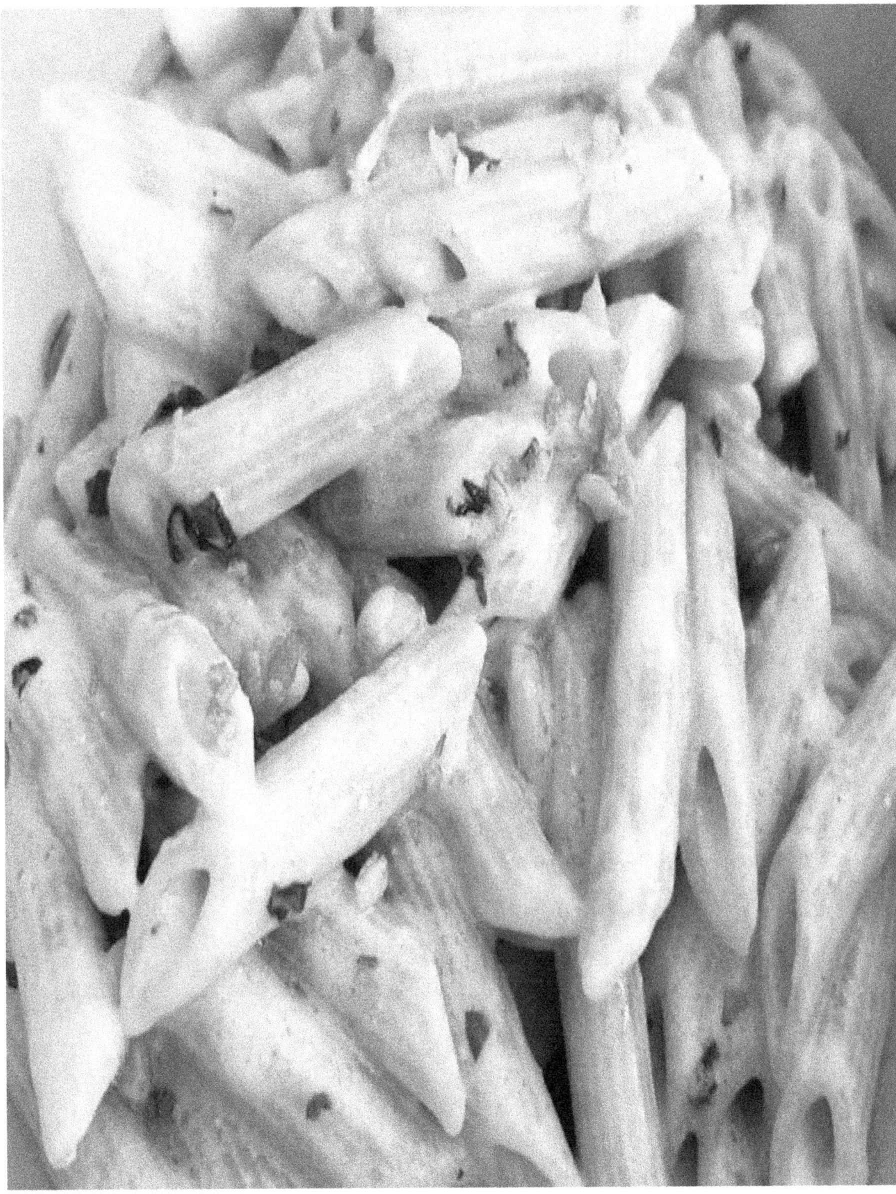

Prep time:

10 minutes | Cook time: 11 minutes | Serves 4 to 6

Ingredients

8 ounces (227 g) spaghetti

4 tablespoons almond butter

1 teaspoon freshly ground black pepper

½ cup pine nuts

1 cup fresh grated Parmesan cheese, divided

Direction

1. Bring a large pot of salted water to a boil. Add the pasta and cook for 8 minutes.
2. In a large saucepan over medium heat, combine the butter, black pepper, and pine nuts. Cook for 2 to 3 minutes, or until the pine nuts are lightly toasted.
3. Reserve ½ cup of the pasta water. Drain the pasta and place it into the pan with the pine nuts.
4. Add ¾ cup of the Parmesan cheese and the reserved pasta water to the pasta and toss everything together to evenly coat the pasta.
5. Transfer the pasta to a serving dish and top with the remaining ¼ cup of the Parmesan cheese. Serve immediately.

Per Serving

Calories: 542 | fat: 32.0g | protein: 20.0g | carbs: 46.0g | fiber: 2.0g | sodium: 552mg

Creamy Garlic Parmesan Chicken Pasta

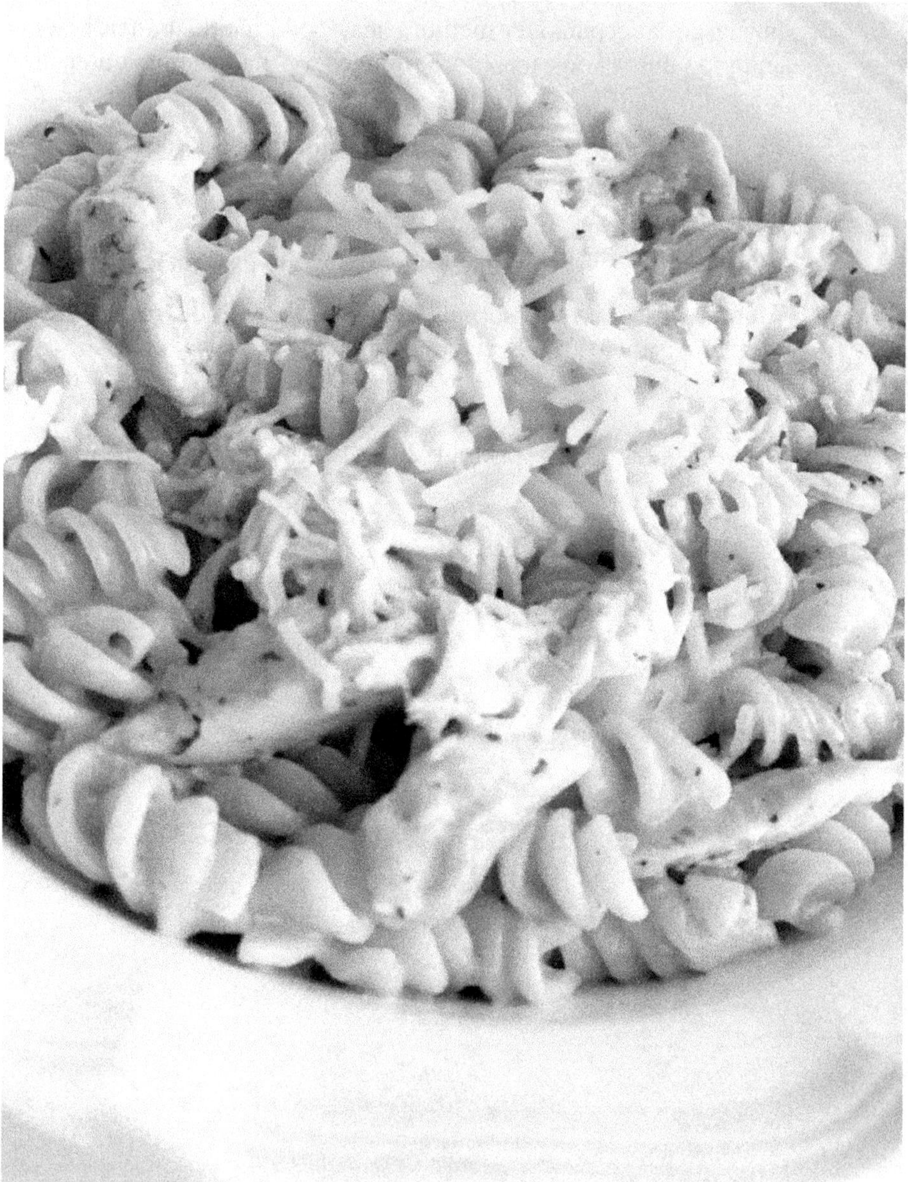

Prep time:

5 minutes | Cook time: 15 minutes | Serves 4

Ingredients

3 tablespoons extra-virgin olive oil

2 boneless, skinless chicken breasts, cut into thin strips

1 large onion, thinly sliced

3 tablespoons garlic, minced

1½ teaspoons salt

1 pound (454 g) fettuccine pasta

1 cup heavy whipping cream

¾ cup freshly grated Parmesan cheese, divided

½ teaspoon freshly ground black pepper

Direction

1. In a large skillet over medium heat, heat the olive oil. Add the chicken and cook for 3 minutes.
2. Add the onion, garlic and salt to the skillet. Cook for 7 minutes, stirring occasionally.
3. Meanwhile, bring a large pot of salted water to a boil and add the pasta, then cook for 7 minutes.
4. While the pasta is cooking, add the heavy cream, ½ cup of the Parmesan cheese and black pepper to the chicken. Simmer for 3 minutes.
5. Reserve ½ cup of the pasta water. Drain the pasta and add it to the chicken cream sauce.
6. Add the reserved pasta water to the pasta and toss together. Simmer for 2 minutes. Top with the remaining ¼ cup of the Parmesan cheese and serve warm.

Per Serving

Calories: 879 | fat: 42.0g | protein: 35.0g | carbs: 90.0g | fiber: 5.0g | sodium: 1336mg

Bulgur Pilaf with Garbanzo

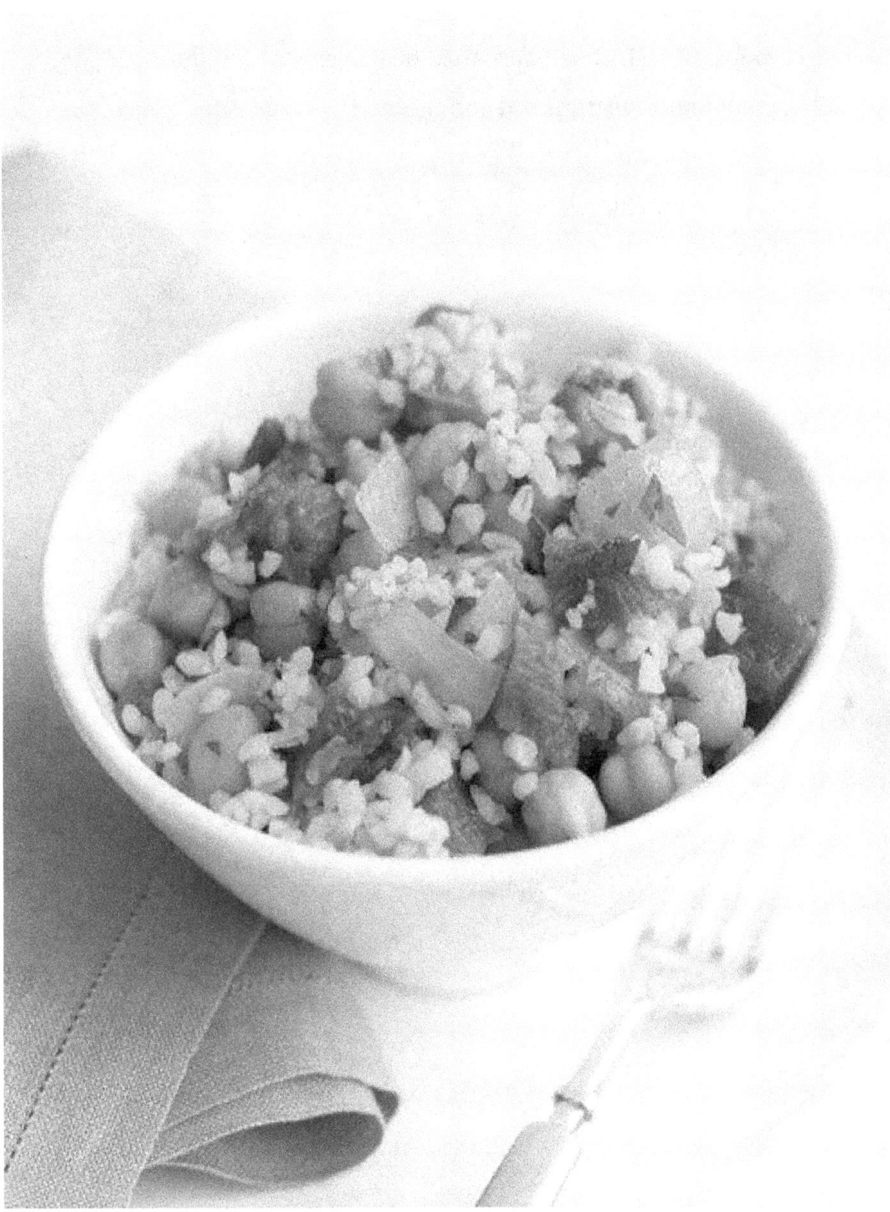

Prep time:

5 minutes | Cook time: 20 minutes | Serves 4 to 6

Ingredients

3 tablespoons extra-virgin olive oil

1 large onion, chopped

1 (1-pound / 454-g) can garbanzo beans, rinsed and drained

2 cups bulgur wheat, rinsed and drained

1½ teaspoons salt

½ teaspoon cinnamon

4 cups water

Direction

1. In a large pot over medium heat, heat the olive oil. Add the onion and cook for 5 minutes.
2. Add the garbanzo beans and cook for an additional 5 minutes.
3. Stir in the remaining Ingredients.
4. Reduce the heat to low. Cover and cook for 10 minutes.
5. When done, fluff the pilaf with a fork. Cover and let sit for another 5 minutes before serving.

Per Serving

Calories: 462 | fat: 13.0g | protein: 15.0g | carbs: 76.0g | fiber: 19.0g | sodium: 890mg

Pearl Barley Risotto with Parmesan Cheese

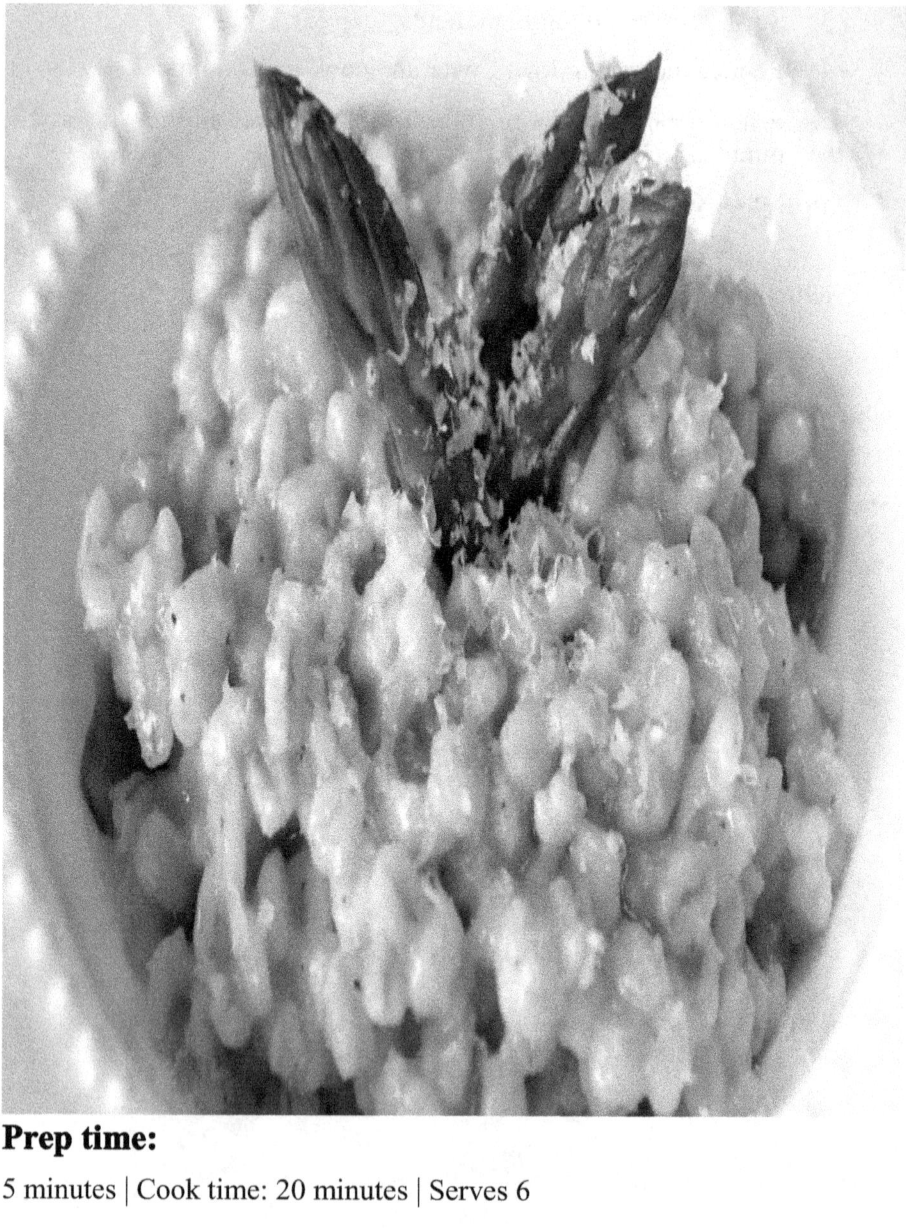

Prep time:

5 minutes | Cook time: 20 minutes | Serves 6

Ingredients

4 cups low-sodium or no-salt-added vegetable broth

1 tablespoon extra-virgin olive oil

1 cup chopped yellow onion

2 cups uncooked pearl barley

½ cup dry white wine

1 cup freshly grated Parmesan cheese, divided

¼ teaspoon kosher or sea salt

¼ teaspoon freshly ground black pepper

Fresh chopped chives and lemon wedges, for serving (optional)

Direction

1. Pour the broth into a medium saucepan and bring to a simmer.
2. Heat the olive oil in a large stockpot over medium-high heat. Add the onion and cook for about 4 minutes, stirring occasionally.
3. Add the barley and cook for 2 minutes, stirring, or until the barley is toasted. Pour in the wine and cook for about 1 minute, or until most of the liquid evaporates. Add 1 cup of the warm broth into the pot and cook, stirring, for about 2 minutes, or until most of the liquid is absorbed.
4. Add the remaining broth, 1 cup at a time, cooking until each cup is absorbed (about 2 minutes each time) before adding the next. The last addition of broth will take a bit longer to absorb, about 4 minutes.
5. Remove the pot from the heat, and stir in ½ cup of the cheese, and the salt and pepper.
6. Serve with the remaining ½ cup of the cheese on the side, along with the chives and lemon wedges (if desired).

Per Serving

Calories: 421 | fat: 11.0g | protein: 15.0g | carbs: 67.0g | fiber: 11.0g | sodium: 641mg

Israeli Couscous with Asparagus

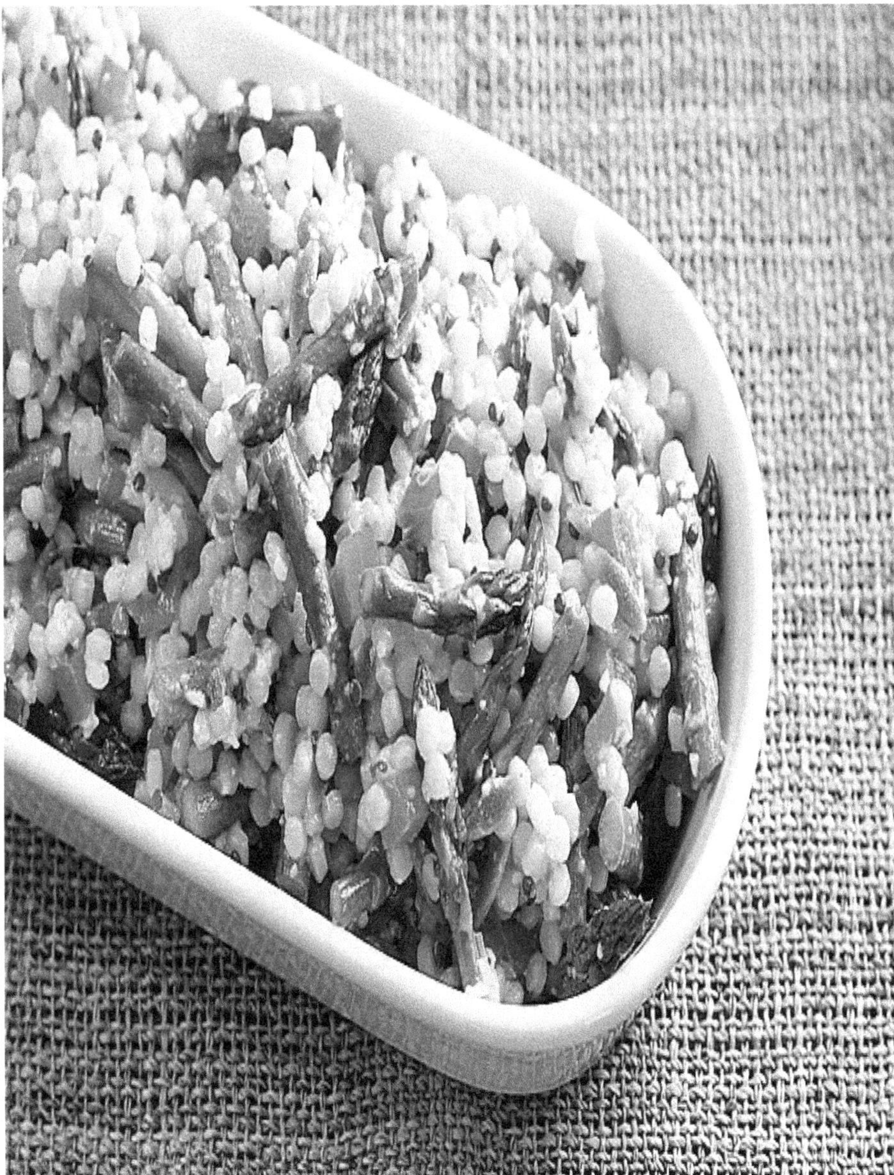

Prep time:

5 minutes | Cook time: 25 minutes | Serves 6

Ingredients

1½ pounds (680 g) asparagus spears, ends trimmed and stalks chopped into 1-inch pieces

1 garlic clove, minced

1 tablespoon extra-virgin olive oil

¼ teaspoon freshly ground black pepper

1¾ cups water

1 (8-ounce / 227-g) box uncooked whole-wheat or regular

Israeli couscous

(about 1⅓ cups)

¼ teaspoon kosher salt

1 cup garlic-and-herb goat cheese, at room temperature

Direction

1. Preheat the oven to 425ºF (220ºC).
2. In a large bowl, stir together the asparagus, garlic, oil, and pepper. Spread the asparagus on a large, rimmed baking sheet and roast for 10 minutes, stirring a few times. Remove the pan from the oven, and spoon the asparagus into a large serving bowl. Set aside.
3. While the asparagus is roasting, bring the water to a boil in a medium saucepan. Add the couscous and season with salt, stirring well.
4. Reduce the heat to medium-low. Cover and cook for 12 minutes, or until the water is absorbed.
5. Pour the hot couscous into the bowl with the asparagus. Add the goat cheese and mix thoroughly until completely melted.
6. Serve immediately.

Per Serving

Calories: 103 | fat: 2.0g | protein: 6.0g | carbs: 18.0g | fiber: 5.0g | sodium: 343mg

Freekeh Pilaf with Dates and Pistachios

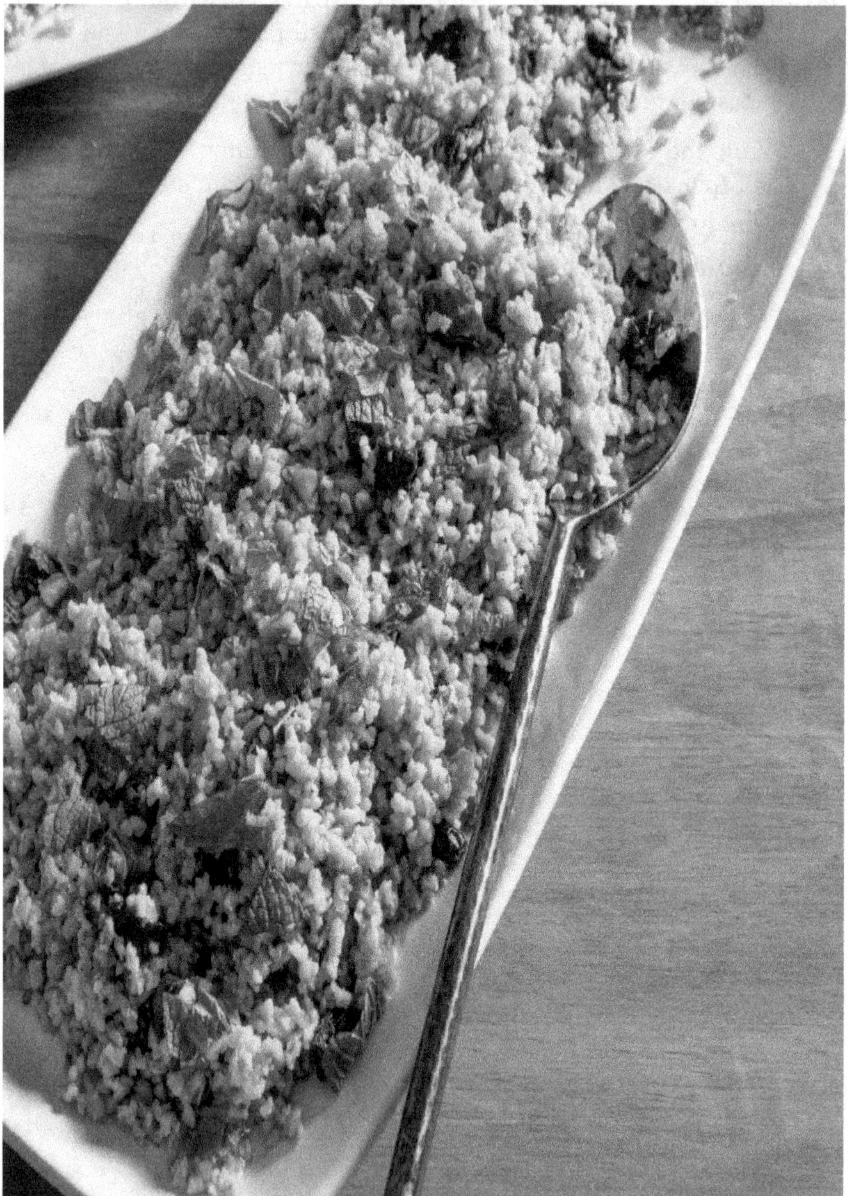

Prep time:

10 minutes | Cook time: 10 minutes | Serves 4 to 6

Ingredients

2 tablespoons extra-virgin olive oil, plus extra for drizzling

1 shallot, minced

1½ teaspoons grated fresh ginger

¼ teaspoon ground coriander

¼ teaspoon ground cumin Salt and pepper, to taste

1¾ cups water

1½ cups cracked freekeh, rinsed

3 ounces (85 g) pitted dates, chopped

¼ cup shelled pistachios, toasted and coarsely chopped

1½ tablespoons lemon juice

¼ cup chopped fresh mint

Direction

1. Set the Instant Pot to Sauté mode and heat the olive oil until shimmering.
2. Add the shallot, ginger, coriander, cumin, salt, and pepper to the pot and cook for about 2 minutes, or until the shallot is softened. Stir in the water and freekeh.
3. Secure the lid. Select the Manual mode and set the cooking time for 4 minutes at High Pressure. Once cooking is complete, do a quick pressure release. Carefully open the lid.
4. Add the dates, pistachios and lemon juice and gently fluff the freekeh with a fork to combine. Season to taste with salt and pepper.
5. Transfer to a serving dish and sprinkle with the mint. Serve drizzled with extra olive oil.

Per Serving

Calories: 280 | fat: 8.0g | protein: 8.0g | carbs: 46.0g | fiber: 9.0g | sodium: 200mg

Quinoa with Baby Potatoes and Broccoli

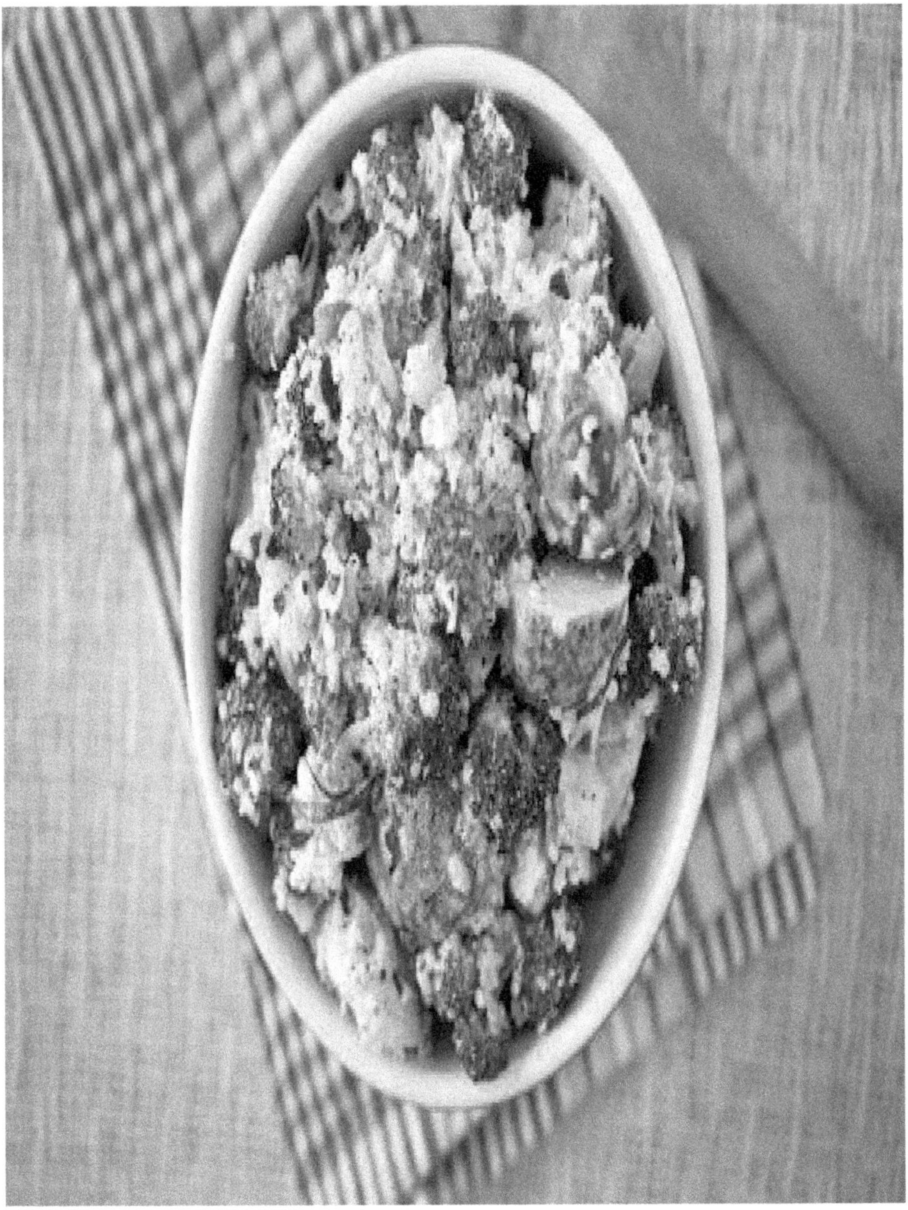

Prep time:

5 minutes | Cook time: 10 minutes | Serves 4

Ingredients

2 tablespoons olive oil

1 cup baby potatoes, cut in half

1 cup broccoli florets

2 cups cooked quinoa

Zest of 1 lemon

Sea salt and freshly ground pepper, to taste

Direction

1. Heat the olive oil in a large skillet over medium heat until shimmering.
2. Add the potatoes and cook for about 6 to 7 minutes, or until softened and golden brown. Add the broccoli and cook for about 3 minutes, or until tender.
3. Remove from the heat and add the quinoa and lemon zest. Season with salt and pepper to taste, then serve.

Per Serving

Calories: 205 | fat: 8.6g | protein: 5.1g | carbs: 27.3g | fiber: 3.7g | sodium: 158mg

Black-Eyed Pea and Vegetable Stew

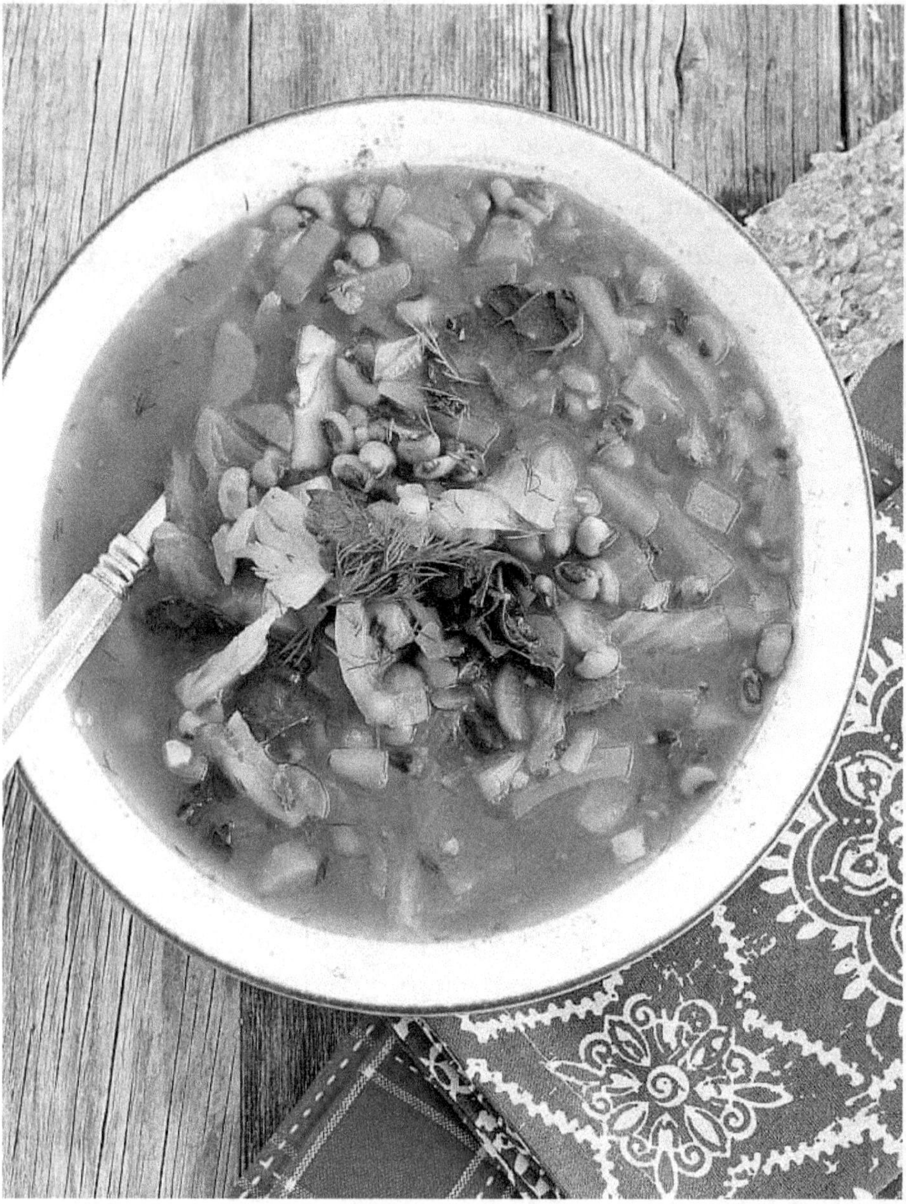

Prep time:

15 minutes | Cook time: 40 minutes | Serves 2

Ingredients

½ cup black-eyed peas, soaked in water overnight

3 cups water, plus more as needed

1 large carrot, peeled and cut into ½-inch pieces (about ¾ cup)

1 large beet, peeled and cut into ½-inch pieces (about ¾ cup)

¼ teaspoon turmeric

¼ teaspoon cayenne pepper

¼ teaspoon ground cumin seeds, toasted

¼ cup finely chopped parsley

¼ teaspoon salt (optional)

½ teaspoon fresh lime juice

Direction

1. Pour the black-eyed peas and water into a large pot, then cook over medium heat for 25 minutes.
2. Add the carrot and beet to the pot and cook for 10 minutes more, adding more water as needed.
3. Add the turmeric, cayenne pepper, cumin, and parsley to the pot and cook for another 6 minutes, or until the vegetables are softened. Stir the mixture periodically. Season with salt, if desired.
4. Serve drizzled with the fresh lime juice.

Per Serving

Calories: 89 | fat: 0.7g | protein: 4.1g | carbs: 16.6g | fiber: 4.5g | sodium: 367mg

Chickpea Salad with Tomatoes and Basil

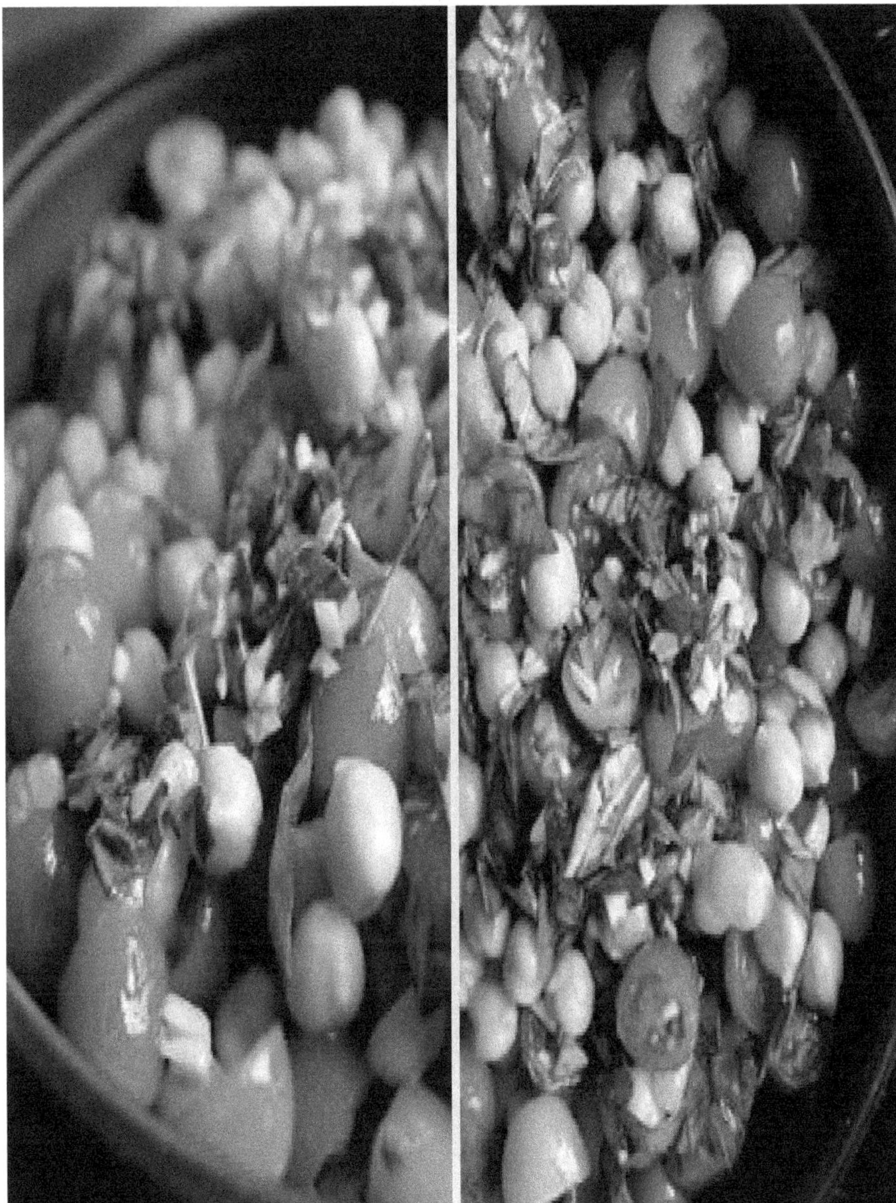

Prep time:

5 minutes | Cook time: 45 minutes | Serves 2

Ingredients

1 cup dried chickpeas, rinsed

1 quart water, or enough to cover the chickpeas by 3 to 4 inches

1½ cups halved grape tomatoes

1 cup chopped fresh basil leaves

2 to 3 tablespoons balsamic vinegar

½ teaspoon garlic powder

½ teaspoon salt, or more to taste

Direction

1. In your Instant Pot, combine the chickpeas and water.
2. Secure the lid. Select the Manual mode and set the cooking time for 45 minutes at High Pressure.
3. Once cooking is complete, do a natural pressure release for 20 minutes, then release any remaining pressure. Carefully open the lid and drain the chickpeas. Refrigerate to cool (unless you want to serve this warm, which is good, too).
4. While the chickpeas cool, in a large bowl, stir together the basil, tomatoes, vinegar, garlic powder, and salt. Add the beans, stir to combine, and serve.

Per Serving

Calories: 395 | fat: 6.0g | protein: 19.8g | carbs: 67.1g | fiber: 19.0g | sodium: 612mg

Mediterranean Lentils

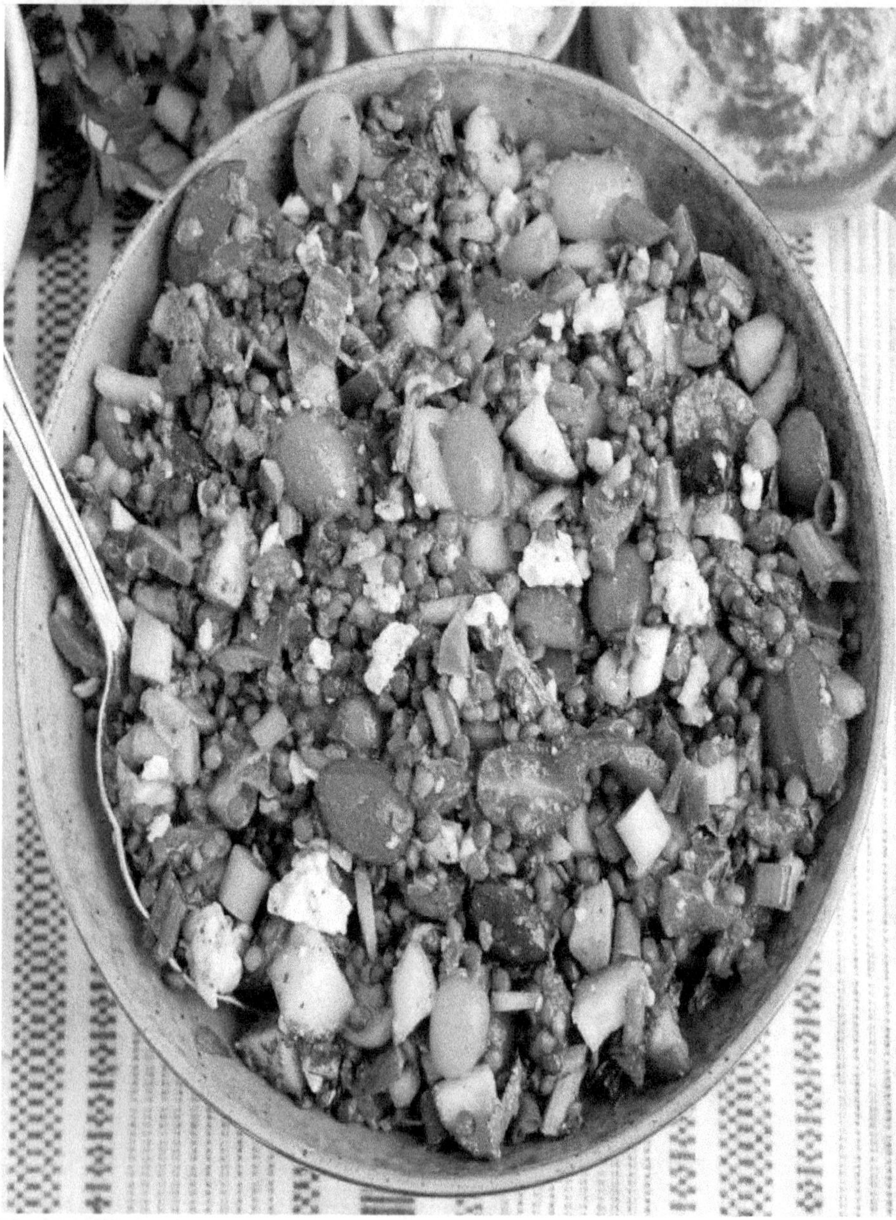

Prep time:

7 minutes | Cook time: 24 minutes | Serves 2

Ingredients

1 tablespoon olive oil

1 small sweet or yellow onion, diced

1 garlic clove, diced

1 teaspoon dried oregano

½ teaspoon ground cumin

½ teaspoon dried parsley

½ teaspoon salt, plus more as needed

¼ teaspoon freshly ground black pepper, plus more as needed

1 tomato, diced

1 cup brown or green lentils

2½ cups vegetable stock

1 bay leaf

Direction

1. Set your Instant Pot to Sauté and heat the olive oil until it shimmers.
2. Add the onion and cook for 3 to 4 minutes until soft. Turn off the Instant Pot and add the garlic, oregano, cumin, parsley, salt, and pepper. Cook until fragrant, about 1 minute.
3. Stir in the tomato, lentils, stock, and bay leaf.
4. Lock the lid. Select the Manual mode and set the cooking time for 18 minutes at High Pressure.
5. When the timer beeps, perform a natural pressure release for 10 minutes, then release any remaining pressure. Carefully open the lid.
6. Remove and discard the bay leaf. Taste and season with more salt and pepper, as needed. If there's too much liquid remaining, select Sauté and cook until it evaporates.
7. Serve warm.

Per Serving

Calories: 426 | fat: 8.1g | protein: 26.2g | carbs: 63.8g | fiber: 31.0g | sodium: 591mg

Mediterranean-Style Beans and Greens

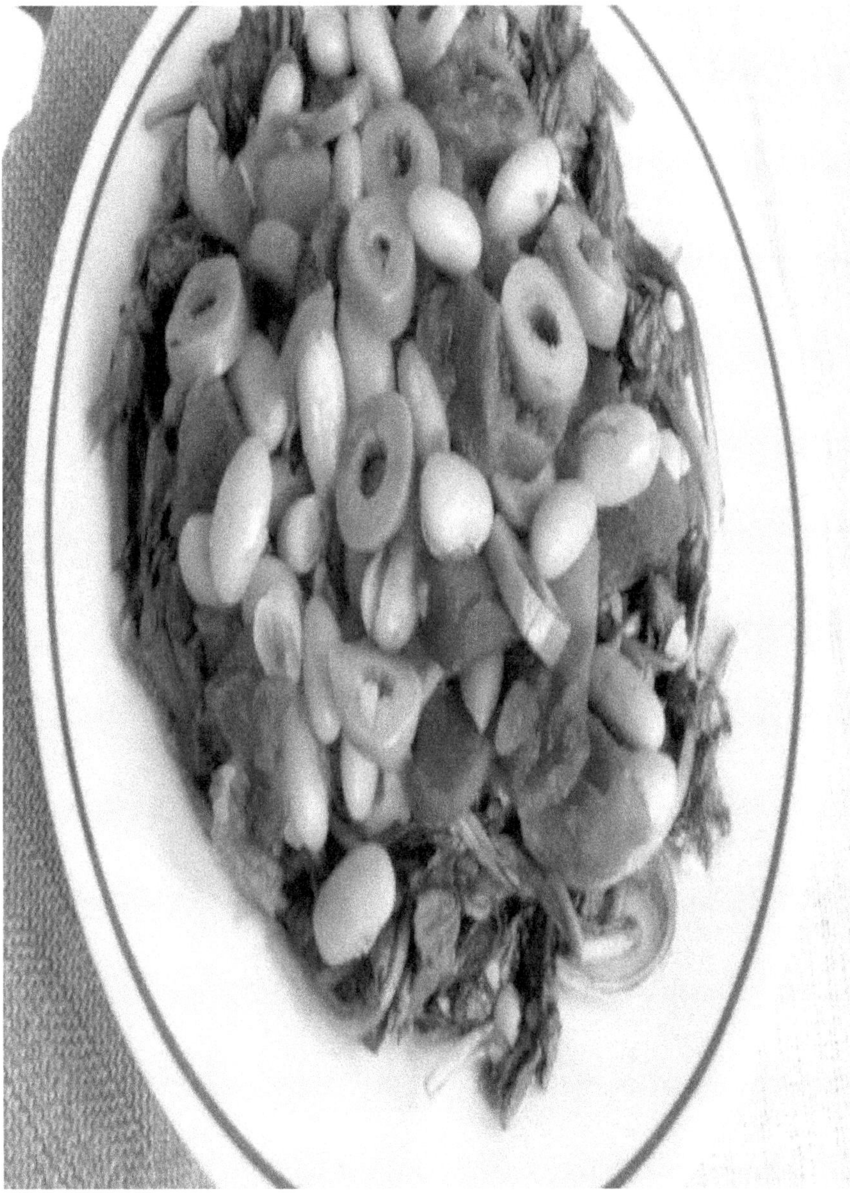

Prep time:

10 minutes | Cook time: 15 minutes | Serves 2

Ingredients

1 (14.5-ounce / 411-g) can diced tomatoes with juice

1 (15-ounce / 425-g) can cannellini beans, drained and rinsed

2 tablespoons chopped green olives, plus 1 or 2 sliced for garnish

¼ cup vegetable broth, plus more as needed

1 teaspoon extra-virgin olive oil

2 cloves garlic, minced

4 cups arugula

¼ cup freshly squeezed lemon juice

Direction

1. In a medium saucepan, bring the tomatoes, beans, and chopped olives to a low boil, adding just enough broth to make the Ingredients saucy (you may need more than ¼ cup if your canned tomatoes don't have a lot of juice). Reduce heat to low and simmer for about 5 minutes.
2. Meanwhile, in a large skillet, heat the olive oil over medium-high heat. When the oil is hot and starts to shimmer, add garlic and sauté just until it starts to turn slightly tan, about 30 seconds. Add the arugula and lemon juice, stirring to coat leaves with the olive oil and juice. Cover, reduce the heat to low, and simmer for 3 to 5 minutes.
3. Serve the beans over the greens and garnish with olive slices.

Per Serving

Calories: 262 | fat: 5.9g | protein: 13.2g | carbs: 40.4g | fiber: 9.8g | sodium: 897mg

Rich Cauliflower Alfredo

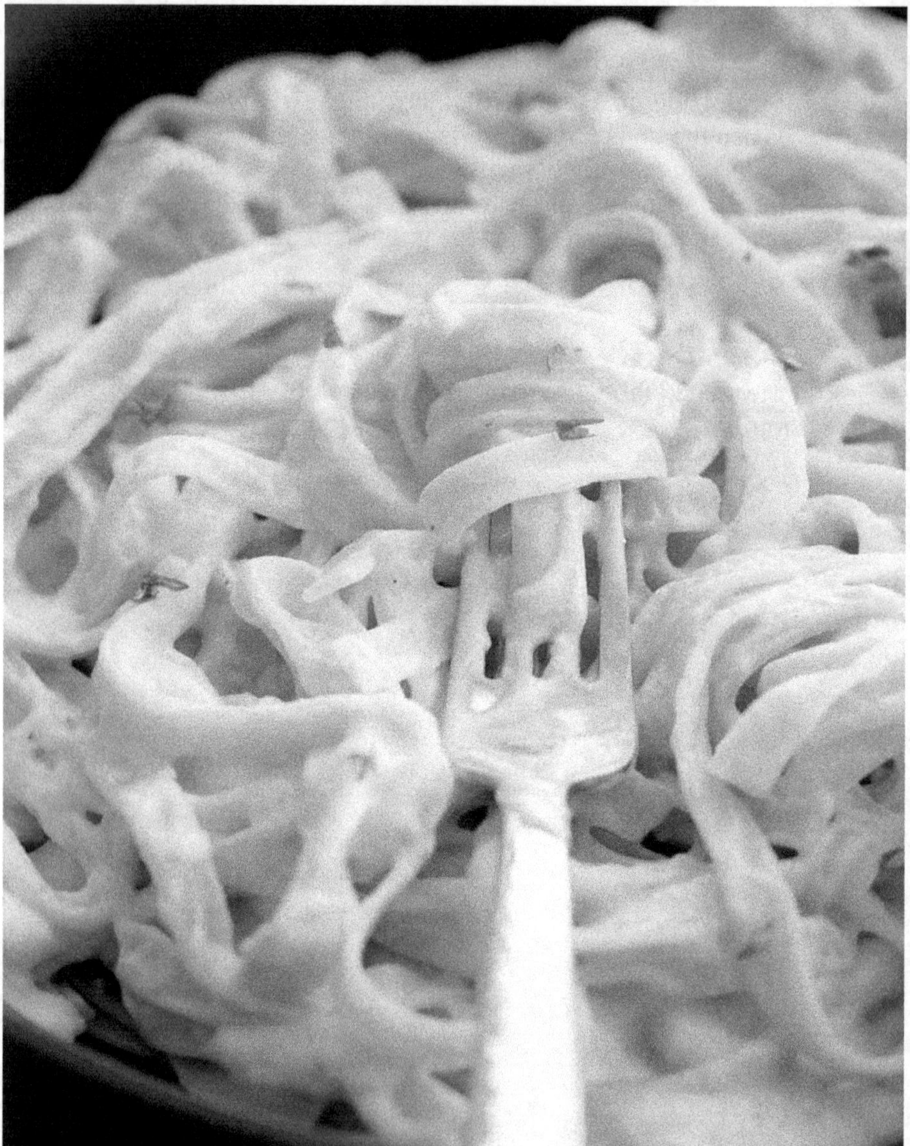

Prep time:

35 minutes | Cook time: 30 minutes | Serves 4

Ingredients

Cauliflower Alfredo Sauce:

1 tablespoon avocado oil

½ yellow onion, diced

2 cups cauliflower florets

2 garlic cloves, minced

1½ teaspoons miso

1 teaspoon Dijon mustard

Pinch of ground nutmeg

½ cup unsweetened almond milk

1½ tablespoons fresh lemon juice

2 tablespoons nutritional yeast

Sea salt and ground black pepper, to taste

Fettuccine:

1 tablespoon avocado oil

½ yellow onion, diced

1 cup broccoli florets

1 zucchini, halved lengthwise and cut into ¼-inch-thick half-moons

Sea salt and ground black pepper, to taste

½ cup sun-dried tomatoes, drained if packed in oil

8 ounces (227 g) cooked whole-wheat fettuccine

½ cup fresh basil, cut into ribbons

Direction

Make the Sauce

1. Heat the avocado oil in a nonstick skillet over medium-high heat until shimmering.
2. Add half of the onion to the skillet and sauté for 5 minutes or until translucent.
3. Add the cauliflower and garlic to the skillet. Reduce the heat to low and cook for 8 minutes or until the cauliflower is tender.
4. Pour them in a food processor, add the remaining Ingredients for the sauce and pulse to combine well. Set aside.

Make the Fettuccine

5. Heat the avocado oil in a nonstick skillet over medium-high heat.
6. Add the remaining half of onion and sauté for 5 minutes or until translucent.
7. Add the broccoli and zucchini. Sprinkle with salt and ground black pepper, then sauté for 5 minutes or until tender.
8. Add the sun-dried tomatoes, reserved sauce, and fettuccine. Sauté for 3 minutes or until well-coated and heated through.
9. Serve the fettuccine on a large plate and spread with basil before serving.

Per Serving

Calories: 288 | fat: 15.9g | protein: 10.1g | carbs: 32.5g | fiber: 8.1g | sodium: 185mg

Butternut Squash and Zucchini with Penne

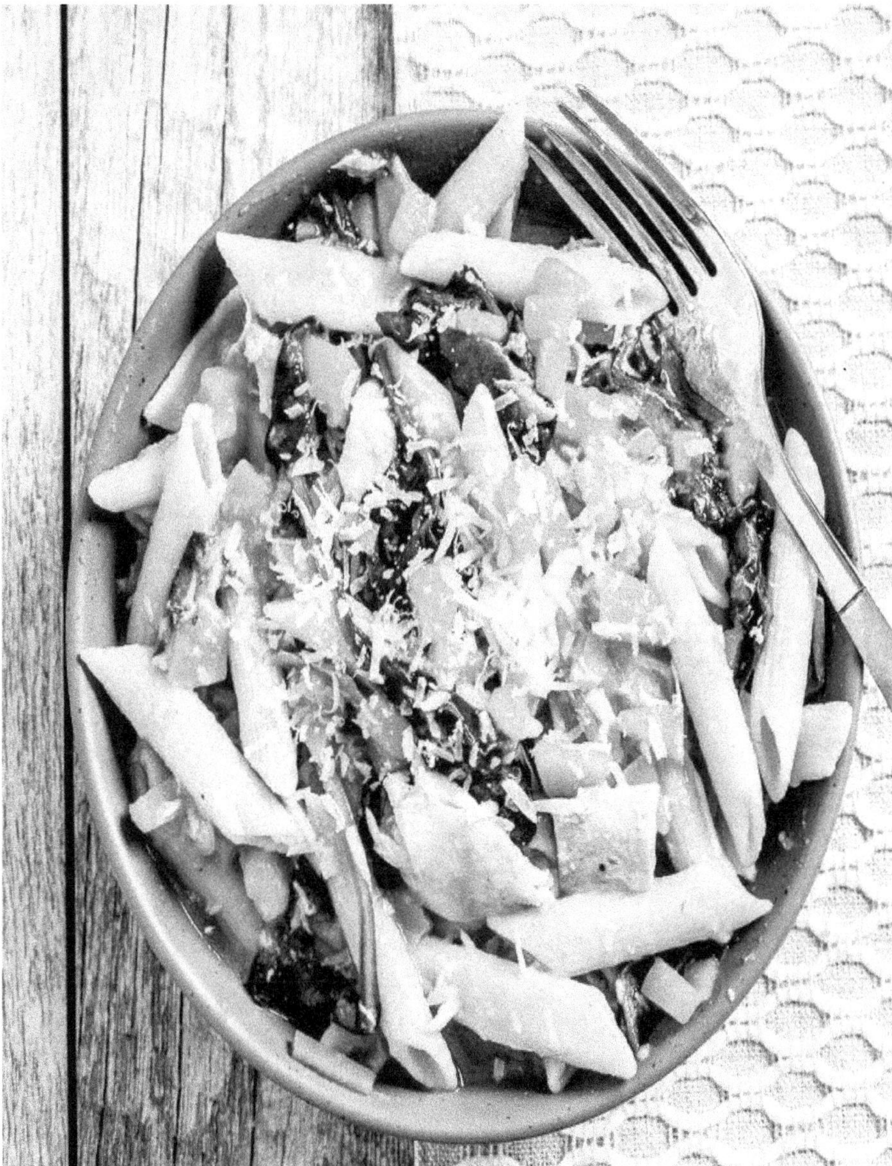

Prep time:

15 minutes | Cook time: 30 minutes | Serves 6

Ingredients

1 large zucchini, diced

1 large butternut squash, peeled and diced

1 large yellow onion, chopped

2 tablespoons extra-virgin olive oil

1 teaspoon paprika

½ teaspoon garlic powder

½ teaspoon sea salt

½ teaspoon freshly ground black pepper

1 pound (454 g) whole-grain penne

½ cup dry white wine

2 tablespoons grated Parmesan cheese

Direction

1. Preheat the oven to 400°F (205°C). Line a baking sheet with aluminum foil.
2. Combine the zucchini, butternut squash, and onion in a large bowl. Drizzle with olive oil and sprinkle with paprika, garlic powder, salt, and ground black pepper. Toss to coat well.
3. Spread the vegetables in the single layer on the baking sheet, then roast in the preheated oven for 25 minutes or until the vegetables are tender.
4. Meanwhile, bring a pot of water to a boil, then add the penne and cook for 14 minutes or until al dente. Drain the penne through a colander.
5. Transfer ½ cup of roasted vegetables in a food processor, then pour in the dry white wine. Pulse until smooth.
6. Pour the puréed vegetables in a nonstick skillet and cook with penne over medium-high heat for a few minutes to heat through.
7. Transfer the penne with the purée on a large serving plate, then spread the remaining roasted vegetables and Parmesan on top before serving.

Per Serving

Calories: 340 | fat: 6.2g | protein: 8.0g | carbs: 66.8g | fiber: 9.1g | sodium: 297mg

Small Pasta and Beans Pot

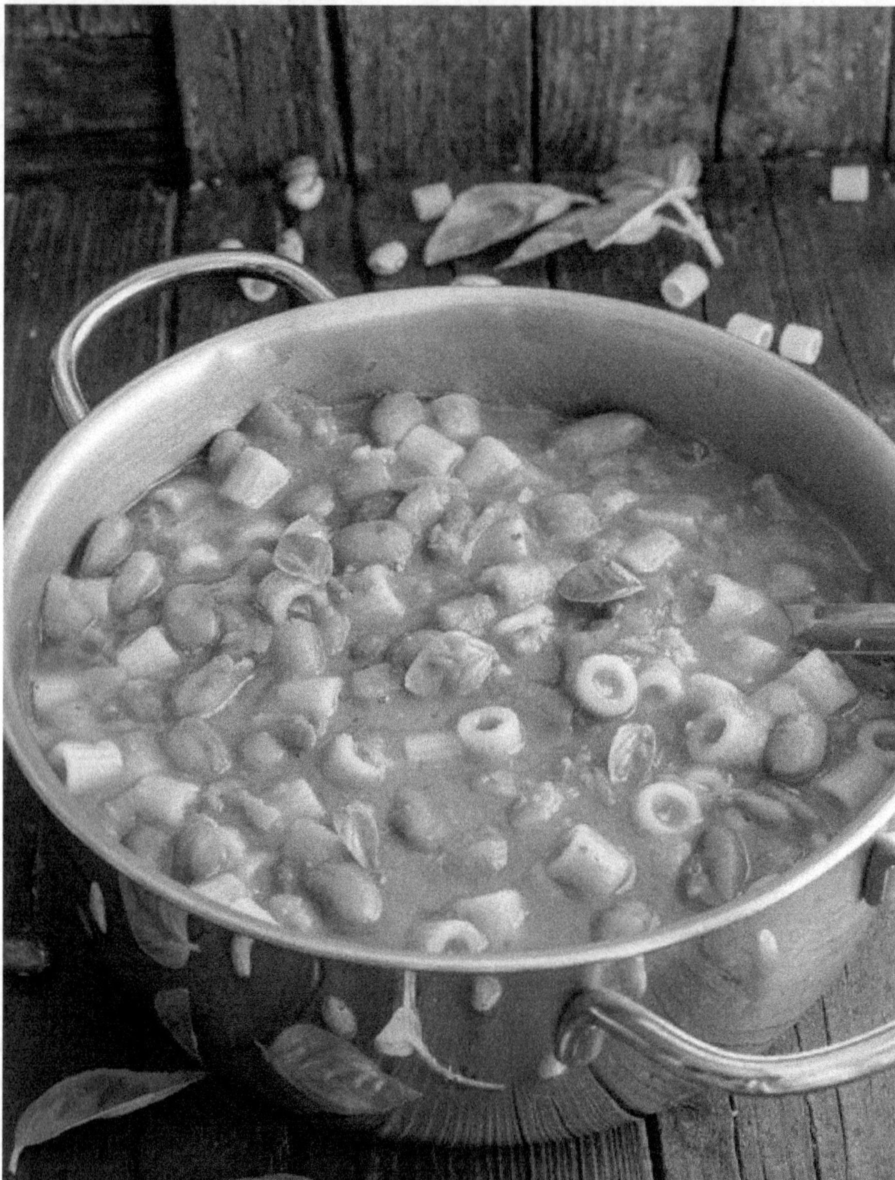

Prep time:

20 minutes | Cook time: 15 minutes | Serves 2 to 4

Ingredients

1 pound (454 g) small whole wheat pasta

1 (14.5-ounce / 411-g) can diced tomatoes, juice reserved

1 (15-ounce / 425-g) can cannellini beans, drained and rinsed

2 tablespoons no-salt-added tomato paste

1 red or yellow bell pepper, chopped

1 yellow onion, chopped

1 tablespoon Italian seasoning mix

3 garlic cloves, minced

¼ teaspoon crushed red pepper flakes, optional

1 tablespoon extra-virgin olive oil

5 cups water

1 bunch kale, stemmed and chopped

½ cup pitted Kalamata olives, chopped

1 cup sliced basil

Direction

1. Except for the kale, olives, and basil, combine all the Ingredients in a pot. Stir to mix well. Bring to a boil over high heat. Stir constantly.
2. Reduce the heat to medium high and add the kale. Cook for 10 minutes or until the pasta is al dente. Stir constantly.
3. Transfer all of them on a large plate and serve with olives and basil on top.

Per Serving

Calories: 357 | fat: 7.6g | protein: 18.2g | carbs: 64.5g | fiber: 10.1g | sodium: 454mg

Swoodles with Almond Butter Sauce

Prep time:

20 minutes | Cook time: 20 minutes | Serves 4

Ingredients

Sauce:

1 garlic clove

1-inch piece fresh ginger, peeled and sliced

¼ cup chopped yellow onion

¾ cup almond butter

1 tablespoon tamari

1 tablespoon raw honey

1 teaspoon paprika

1 tablespoon fresh lemon juice

⅛ teaspoon ground red pepper

Sea salt and ground black pepper, to taste

¼ cup water

Swoodles:

2 large sweet potatoes, spiralized

2 tablespoons coconut oil, melted

Sea salt and ground black pepper, to taste

For Serving:

½ cup fresh parsley, chopped

½ cup thinly sliced scallions

Direction

Make the Sauce

1. Put the garlic, ginger, and onion in a food processor, then pulse to combine well.
2. Add the almond butter, tamari, honey, paprika, lemon juice, ground red pepper, salt, and black pepper to the food processor. Pulse to combine well. Pour in the water during the pulsing until the mixture is thick and smooth.

Make the Swoodles

3. Preheat the oven to 425°F (220°C). Line a baking sheet with parchment paper.
4. Put the spiralized sweet potato in a bowl, then drizzle with olive oil. Toss to coat well. Transfer them on the baking sheet. Sprinkle with salt and pepper.
5. Bake in the preheated oven for 20 minutes or until lightly browned and al dente. Check the doneness during the baking and remove any well-cooked swoodles.
6. Transfer the swoodles on a large plate and spread with sauce, parsley, and scallions. Toss to serve.

Per Serving

Calories: 441 | fat: 33.6g | protein: 12.0g | carbs: 29.6g | fiber: 7.8g | sodium: 479mg

Tomato Sauce and Basil Pesto Fettuccine

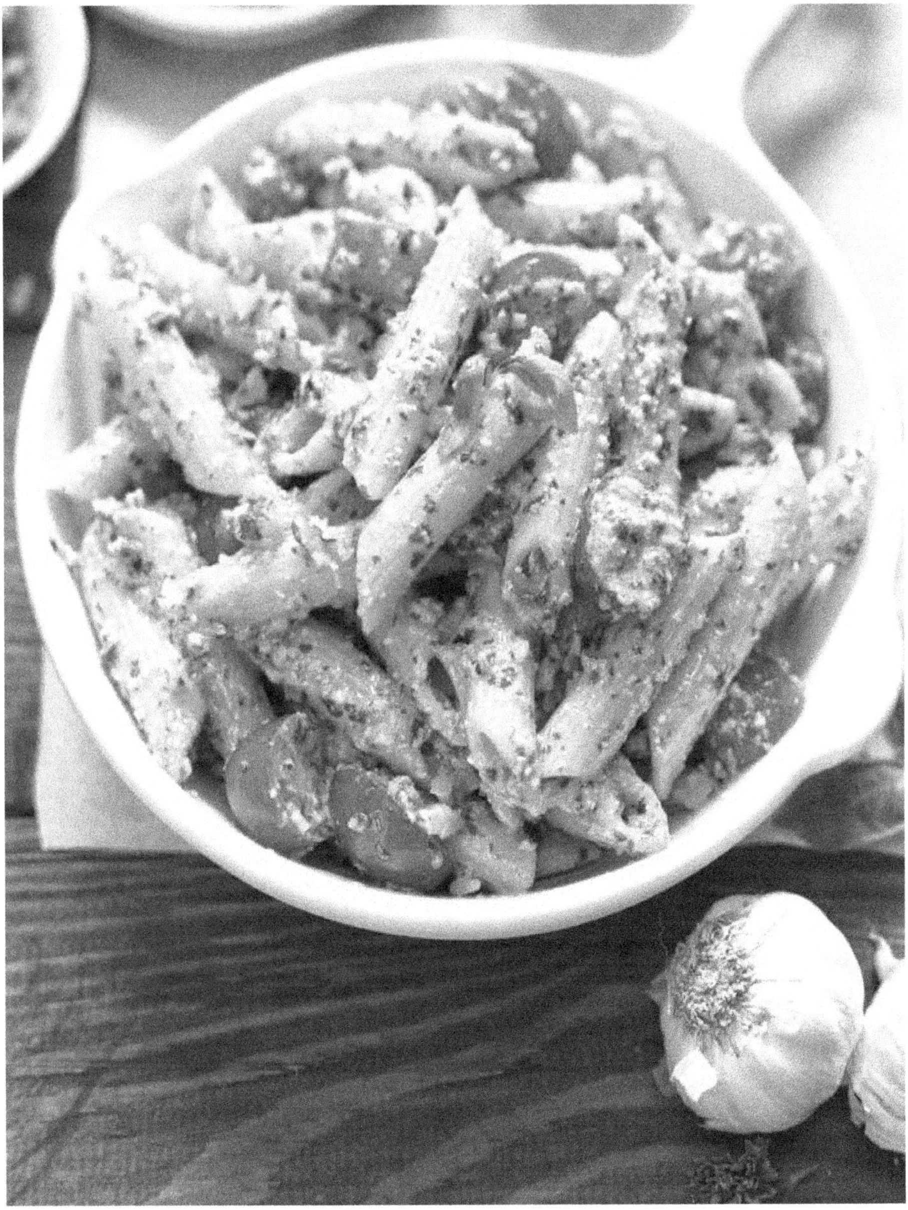

Prep time:

15 minutes | Cook time: 15 minutes | Serves 4

Ingredients

4 Roma tomatoes, diced

2 teaspoons no-salt-added tomato paste

1 tablespoon chopped fresh oregano

2 garlic cloves, minced

1 cup low-sodium vegetable soup

½ teaspoon sea salt

1 packed cup fresh basil leaves

¼ cup pine nuts

¼ cup grated Parmesan cheese

2 tablespoons extra-virgin olive oil

1 pound (454 g) cooked whole-grain fettuccine

Direction

1. Put the tomatoes, tomato paste, oregano, garlic, vegetable soup, and salt in a skillet. Stir to mix well.
2. Cook over medium heat for 10 minutes or until lightly thickened.
3. Put the remaining Ingredients, except for the fettuccine, in a food processor and pulse to combine until smooth.
4. Pour the puréed basil mixture into the tomato mixture, then add the fettuccine. Cook for a few minutes or until heated through and the fettuccine is well coated.
5. Serve immediately.

Per Serving

Calories: 389 | fat: 22.7g | protein: 9.7g | carbs: 40.2g | fiber: 4.8g | sodium: 616mg

Broccoli and Carrot Pasta Salad

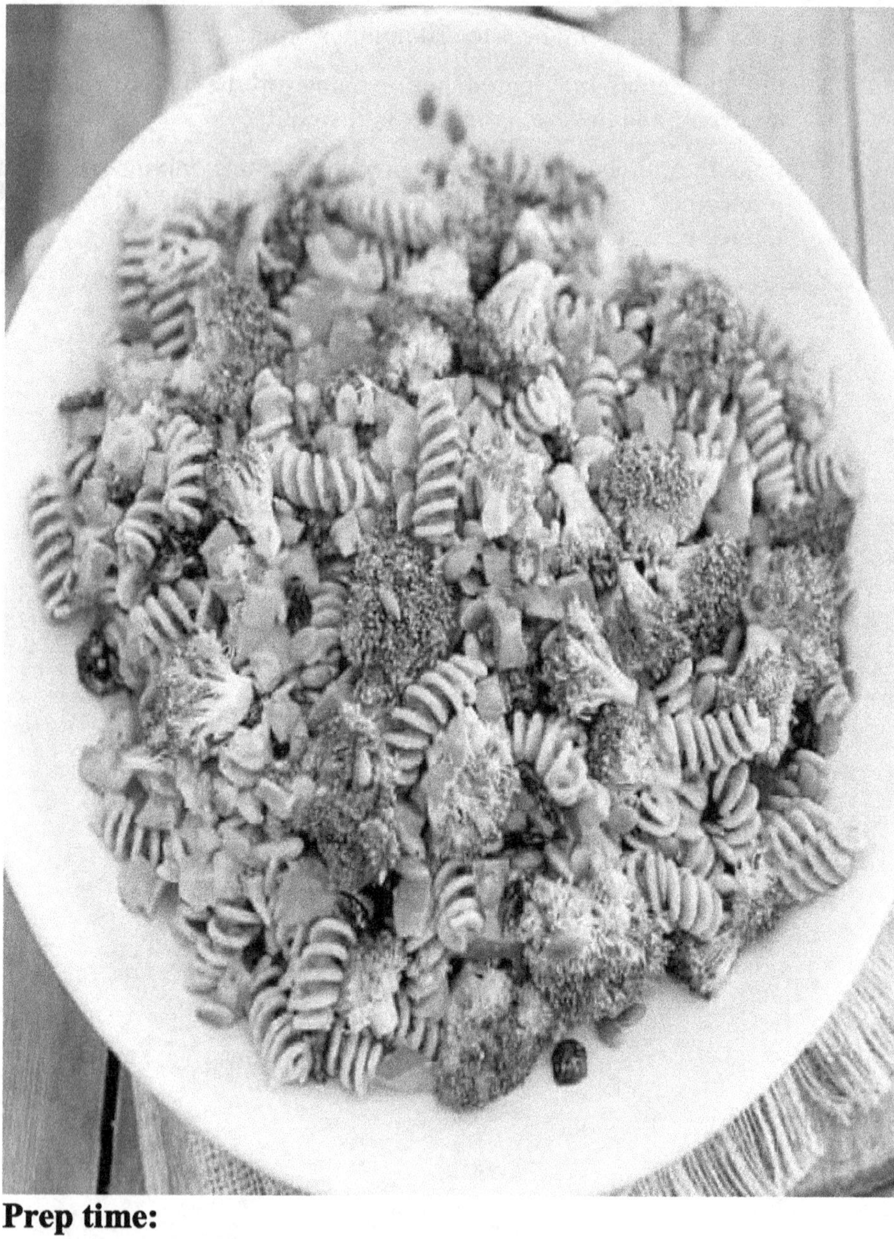

Prep time:

5 minutes | Cook time: 10 minutes | Serves 2

Ingredients

8 ounces (227 g) whole-wheat pasta

2 cups broccoli florets

1 cup peeled and shredded carrots

¼ cup plain Greek yogurt

Juice of 1 lemon

1 teaspoon red pepper flakes

Sea salt and freshly ground pepper, to taste

Direction

1. Bring a large pot of lightly salted water to a boil. Add the pasta to the boiling water and cook until al dente, about 8 to 10 minutes. Drain the pasta and let rest for a few minutes.
2. When cooled, combine the pasta with the veggies, yogurt, lemon juice, and red pepper flakes in a large bowl, and stir thoroughly to combine.
3. Taste and season to taste with salt and pepper. Serve immediately.

Per Serving

Calories: 428 | fat: 2.9g | protein: 15.9g | carbs: 84.6g | fiber: 11.7g | sodium: 642mg

Bean and Veggie Pasta

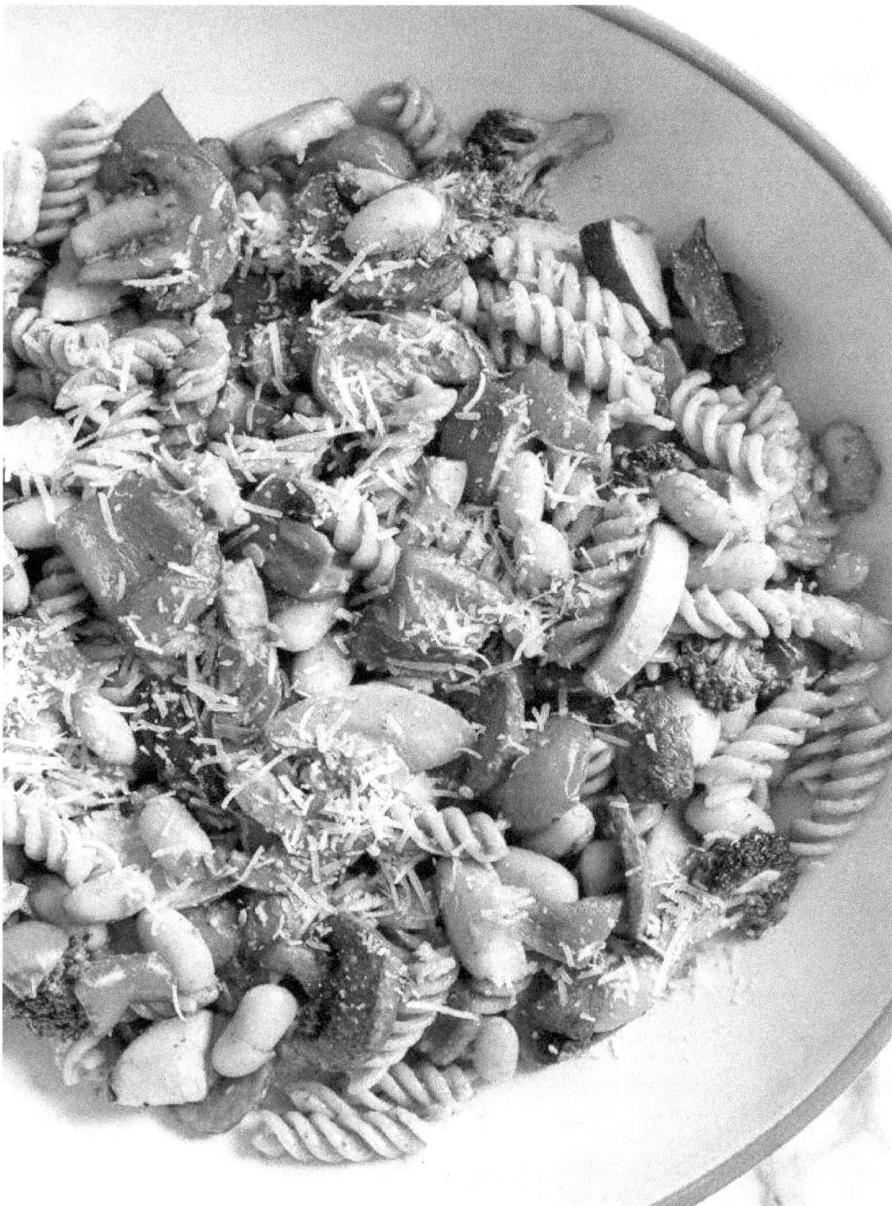

Prep time:

10 minutes | Cook time: 15 minutes | Serves 2

Ingredients

16 ounces (454 g) small whole wheat pasta, such as penne, farfalle, or macaroni

5 cups water

1 (15-ounce / 425-g) can cannellini beans, drained and rinsed

1 (14.5-ounce / 411-g) can diced (with juice) or crushed tomatoes

1 yellow onion, chopped

1 red or yellow bell pepper, chopped

2 tablespoons tomato paste

1 tablespoon olive oil

3 garlic cloves, minced

¼ teaspoon crushed red pepper (optional)

1 bunch kale, stemmed and chopped

1 cup sliced basil

½ cup pitted Kalamata olives, chopped

Direction

1. Add the pasta, water, beans, tomatoes (with juice if using diced), onion, bell pepper, tomato paste, oil, garlic, and crushed red pepper (if desired), to a large stockpot. Bring to a boil over high heat, stirring often.
2. Reduce the heat to medium-high, add the kale, and cook, continuing to stir often, until the pasta is al dente, about 10 minutes.
3. Remove from the heat and let sit for 5 minutes. Garnish with the basil and olives and serve.

Per Serving

Calories: 565 | fat: 17.7g | protein: 18.0g | carbs: 85.5g | fiber: 16.5g | sodium: 540mg

Roasted Ratatouille Pasta

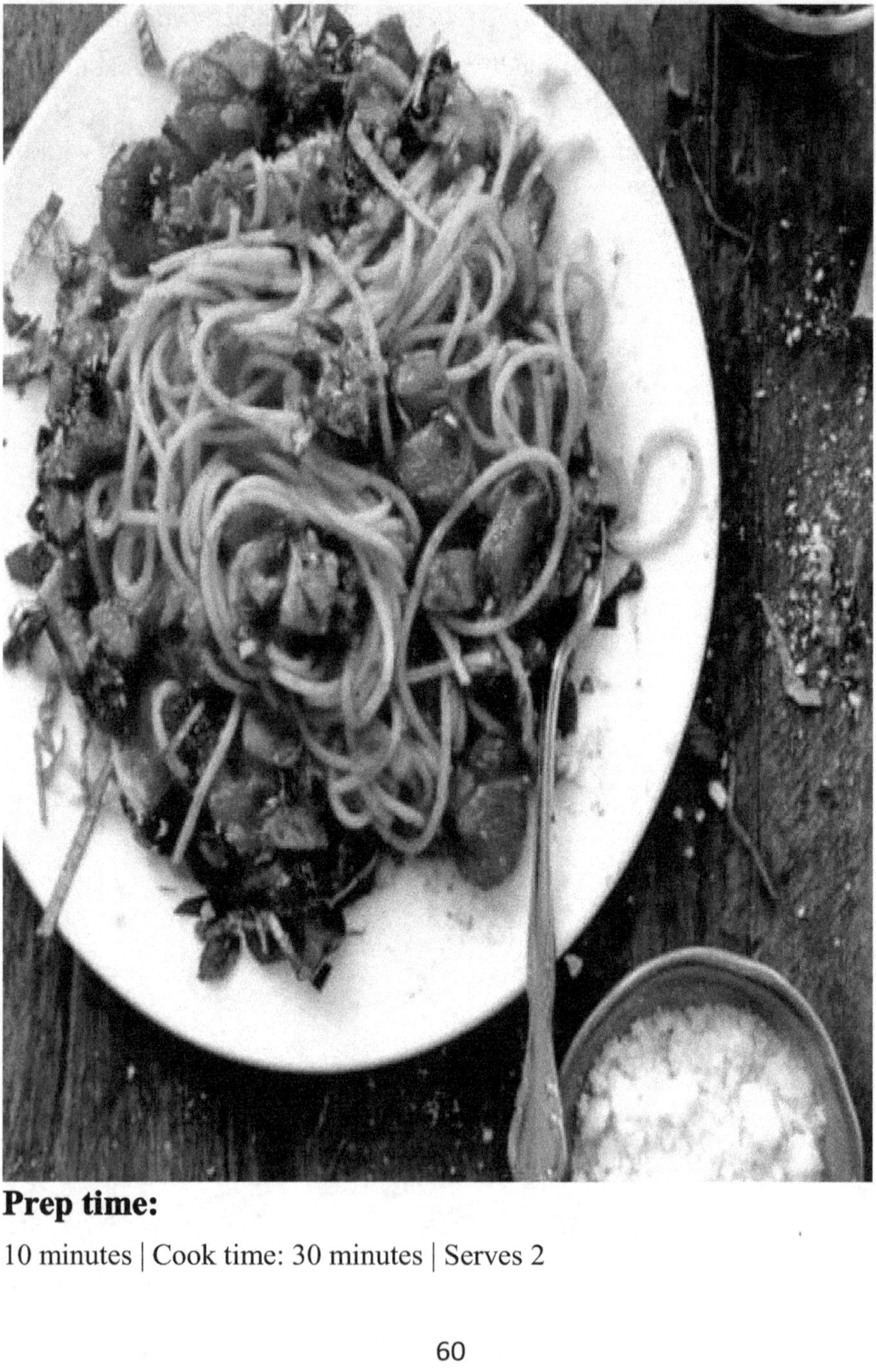

Prep time:

10 minutes | Cook time: 30 minutes | Serves 2

Ingredients

1 small eggplant (about 8 ounces / 227 g)

1 small zucchini

1 portobello mushroom

1 Roma tomato, halved

½ medium sweet red pepper, seeded

½ teaspoon salt, plus additional for the pasta water

1 teaspoon Italian herb seasoning

1 tablespoon olive oil

2 cups farfalle pasta (about 8 ounces / 227 g)

2 tablespoons minced sun-dried tomatoes in olive oil with herbs

2 tablespoons prepared pesto

Direction

1. Slice the ends off the eggplant and zucchini. Cut them lengthwise into ½- inch slices.
2. Place the eggplant, zucchini, mushroom, tomato, and red pepper in a large bowl and sprinkle with ½ teaspoon of salt. Using your hands, toss the vegetables well so that they're covered evenly with the salt. Let them rest for about 10 minutes.
3. While the vegetables are resting, preheat the oven to 400ºF (205ºC). Line a baking sheet with parchment paper.
4. When the oven is hot, drain off any liquid from the vegetables and pat them dry with a paper towel. Add the Italian herb seasoning and olive oil to the vegetables and toss well to coat both sides.
5. Lay the vegetables out in a single layer on the baking sheet. Roast them for 15 to 20 minutes, flipping them over after about 10 minutes or once they start to brown on the underside. When the vegetables are charred in spots, remove them from the oven.
6. While the vegetables are roasting, fill a large saucepan with water. Add salt and cook the pasta until al dente, about 8 to 10 minutes. Drain the pasta, reserving ½ cup of the pasta water.
7. When cool enough to handle, cut the vegetables into large chunks (about 2 inches) and add them to the hot pasta.
8. Stir in the sun-dried tomatoes and pesto and toss everything well. Serve immediately.

Per Serving

Calories: 613 | fat: 16.0g | protein: 23.1g | carbs: 108.5g | fiber: 23.0g | sodium: 775mg

Lentil and Mushroom Pasta

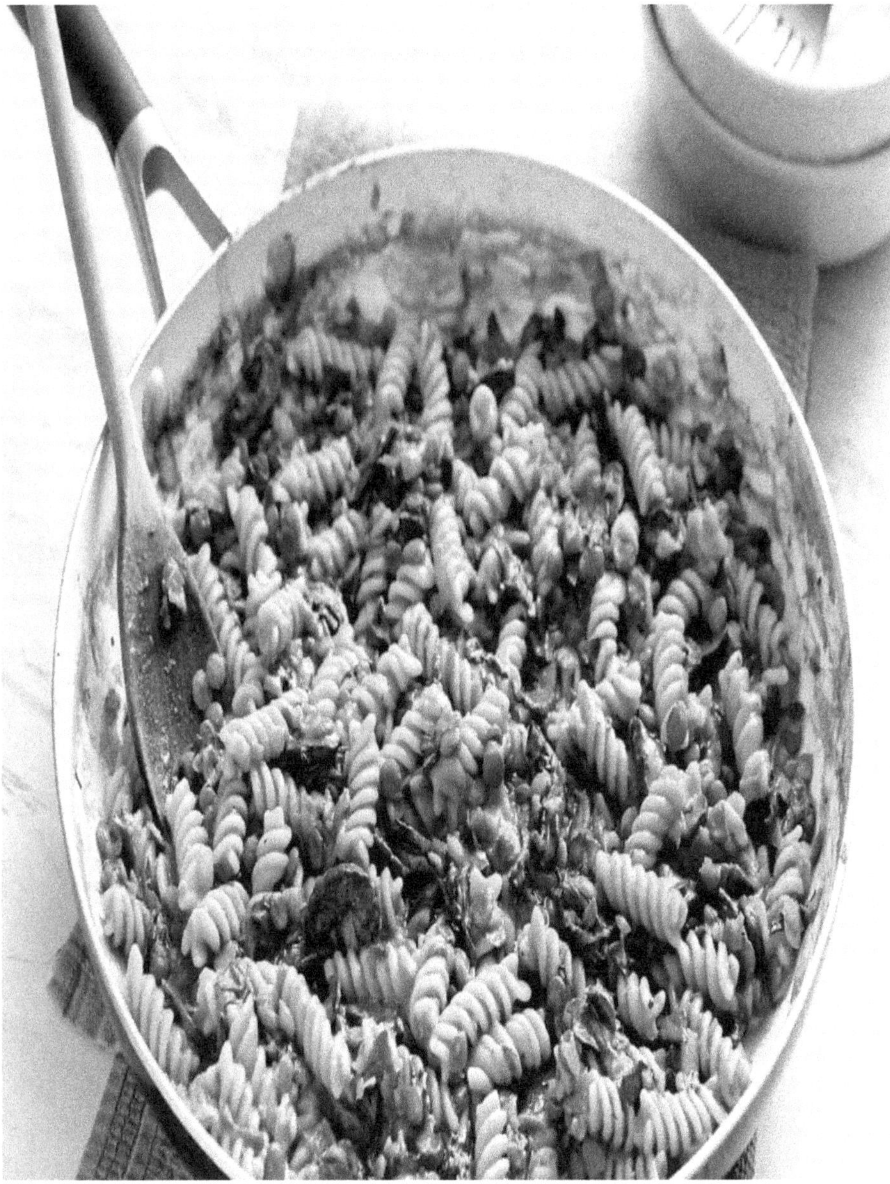

Prep time:

10 minutes | Cook time: 50 minutes | Serves 2

Ingredients

2 tablespoons olive oil

1 large yellow onion, finely diced

2 portobello mushrooms, trimmed and chopped finely

2 tablespoons tomato paste

3 garlic cloves, chopped

1 teaspoon oregano

2½ cups water

1 cup brown lentils

1 (28-ounce / 794-g) can diced tomatoes with basil (with juice if diced)

1 tablespoon balsamic vinegar

Salt and black pepper, to taste

Chopped basil, for garnish

8 ounces (227 g) pasta of choice, cooked

Direction

1. Place a large stockpot over medium heat and add the olive oil. Once the oil is hot, add the onion and mushrooms. Cover and cook until both are soft, about 5 minutes. Add the tomato paste, garlic, and oregano and cook 2 minutes, stirring constantly.
2. Stir in the water and lentils. Bring to a boil, then reduce the heat to medium-low and cook covered for 5 minutes.
3. Add the tomatoes (and juice if using diced) and vinegar. Reduce the heat to low and cook until the lentils are tender, about 30 minutes.
4. Remove from the heat and season with salt and pepper to taste. Garnish with the basil and serve over the cooked pasta.

Per Serving

Calories: 463 | fat: 15.9g | protein: 12.5g | carbs: 70.8g | fiber: 16.9g | sodium: 155mg

Tomato Basil Pasta

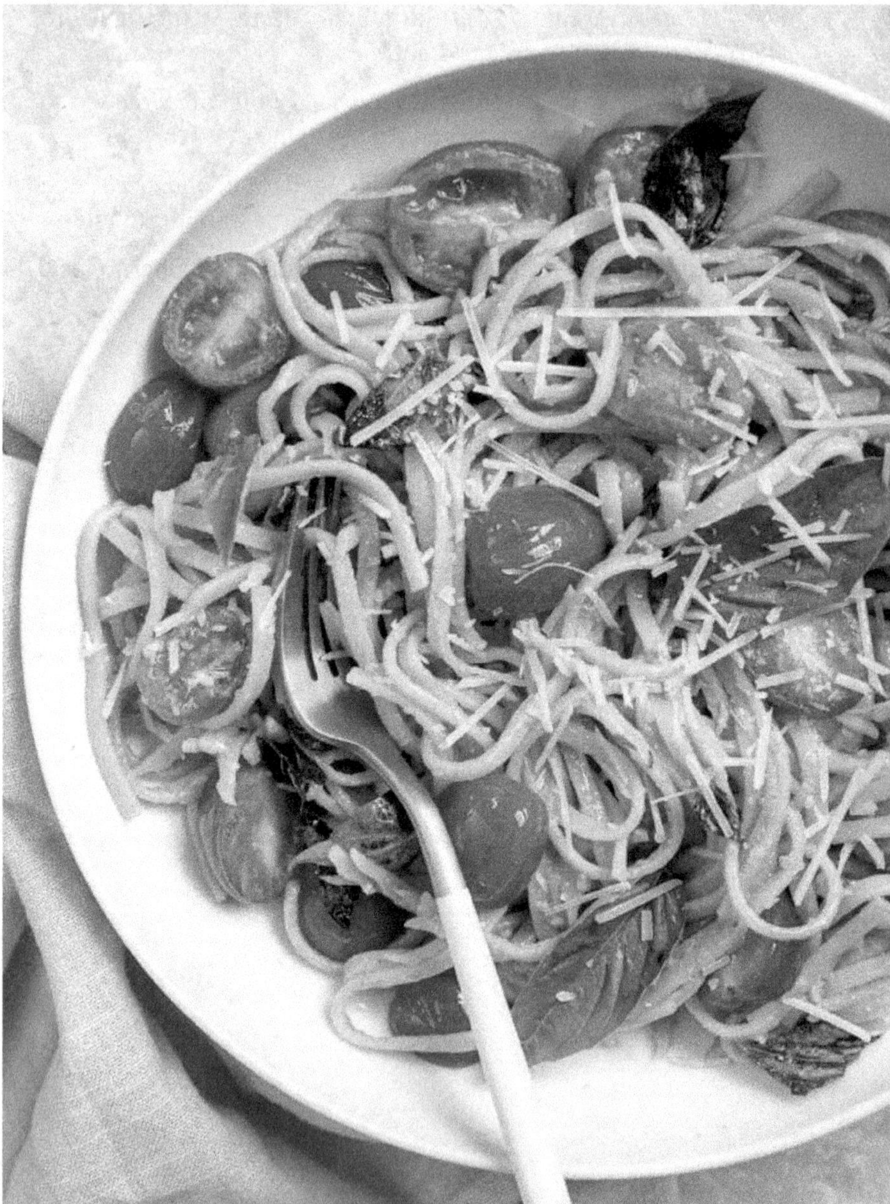

Prep time:

3 minutes | Cook time: 2 minutes | Serves 2

Ingredients

2 cups dried campanelle or similar pasta

1¾ cups vegetable stock

½ teaspoon salt, plus more as needed

2 tomatoes, cut into large dices

1 or 2 pinches red pepper flakes

½ teaspoon garlic powder

½ teaspoon dried oregano

10 to 12 fresh sweet basil leaves

Freshly ground black pepper, to taste

Direction

1. In your Instant Pot, stir together the pasta, stock, and salt. Scatter the tomatoes on top (do not stir).
2. Secure the lid. Select the Manual mode and set the cooking time for 2 minutes at High Pressure.
3. Once cooking is complete, do a quick pressure release. Carefully open the lid.
4. Stir in the red pepper flakes, oregano, and garlic powder. If there's more than a few tablespoons of liquid in the bottom, select Sauté and cook for 2 to 3 minutes until it evaporates.
5. When ready to serve, chiffonade the basil and stir it in. Taste and season with more salt and pepper, as needed. Serve warm.

Per Serving

Calories: 415 | fat: 2.0g | protein: 15.2g | carbs: 84.2g | fiber: 5.0g | sodium: 485mg

Lentil Risotto

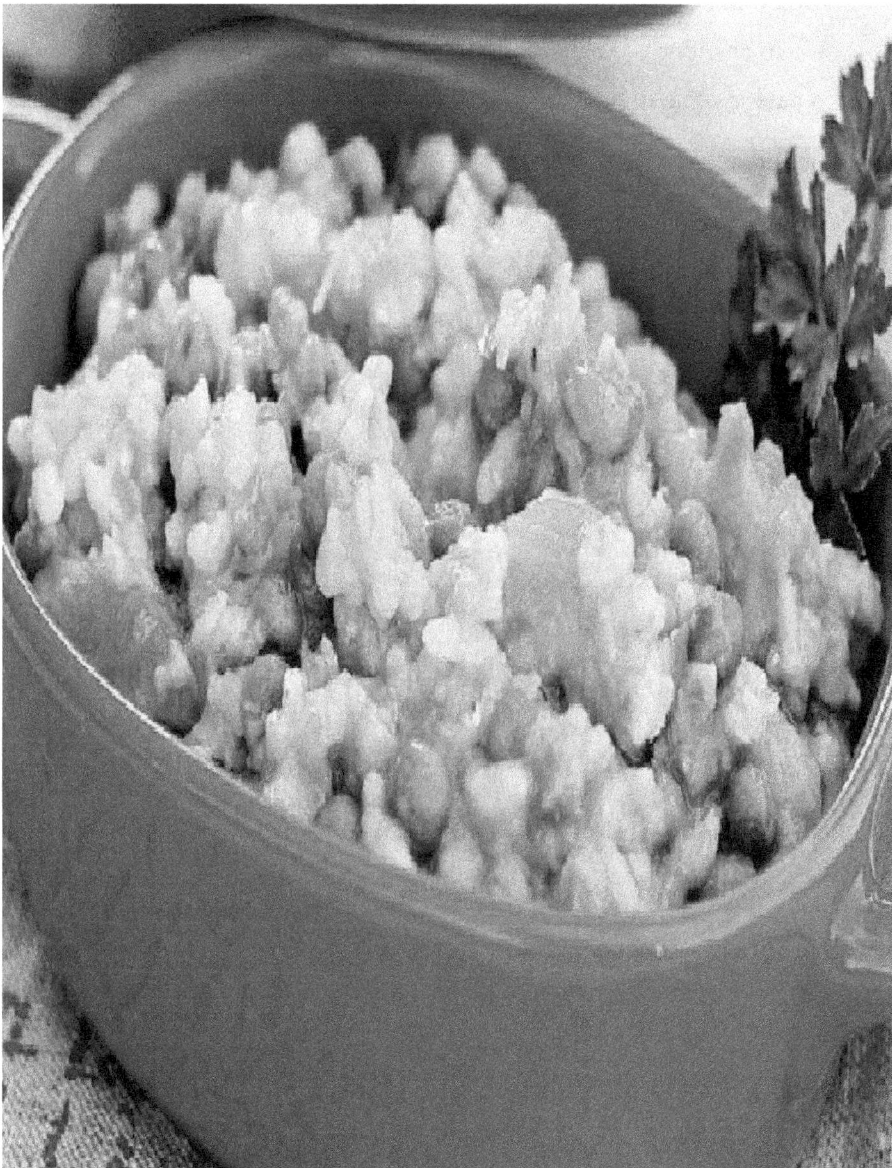

Prep time:

10 minutes | Cook time: 20 minutes | Serves 2

Ingredients

½ tablespoon olive oil

½ medium onion, chopped

½ cup dry lentils, soaked overnight

½ celery stalk, chopped

1 sprig parsley, chopped

½ cup Arborio (short-grain Italian) rice

1 garlic clove, lightly mashed

2 cups vegetable stock

Direction

1. Press the Sauté button to heat your Instant Pot.
2. Add the oil and onion to the Instant Pot and sauté for 5 minutes.
3. Add the remaining Ingredients to the Instant Pot, stirring well.
4. Secure the lid. Select the Manual mode and set the cooking time for 15 minutes at High Pressure.
5. Once cooking is complete, do a natural pressure release for 20 minutes, then release any remaining pressure. Carefully open the lid.
6. Stir and serve hot.

Per Serving

Calories: 261 | fat: 3.6g | protein: 10.6g | carbs: 47.1g | fiber: 8.4g | sodium: 247mg

Bulgur Pilaf with Kale and Tomatoes

Prep time:

10 minutes | Cook time: 10 minutes | Serves 2

Ingredients

2 tablespoons olive oilzxcvn,

2 cloves garlic, minced

1 bunch kale, trimmed and cut into bite-sized pieces

Juice of 1 lemon

2 cups cooked bulgur wheat

1 pint cherry tomatoes, halved

Sea salt and freshly ground pepper, to taste

Direction

1. Heat the olive oil in a large skillet over medium heat. Add the garlic and sauté for 1 minute.
2. Add the kale leaves and stir to coat. Cook for 5 minutes until leaves are cooked through and thoroughly wilted.
3. Add the lemon juice, bulgur and tomatoes. Season with sea salt and freshly ground pepper to taste, then serve.

Per Serving

Calories: 300 | fat: 14.0g | protein: 6.2g | carbs: 37.8g | fiber: 8.7g | sodium: 595mg

Cranberry and Almond Quinoa

Prep time:

5 minutes | Cook time: 10 minutes | Serves 2

Ingredients

2 cups water

1 cup quinoa, rinsed

¼ cup salted sunflower seeds

½ cup slivered almonds

1 cup dried cranberries

Direction

1. Combine water and quinoa in the Instant Pot.
2. Secure the lid. Select the Manual mode and set the cooking time for 10 minutes at High Pressure.
3. Once cooking is complete, do a quick pressure release. Carefully open the lid.
4. Add sunflower seeds, almonds, and dried cranberries and gently mix until well combined.
5. Serve hot.

Per Serving

Calories: 445 | fat: 14.8g | protein: 15.1g | carbs: 64.1g | fiber: 10.2g | sodium: 113mg

Pork and Spinach Spaghetti

Prep time:

15 minutes | Cook time: 16 minutes | Serves 4

Ingredients

2 tablespoons olive oil

½ cup onion, chopped

1 garlic clove, minced

1 pound (454 g) ground pork

2 cups water

1 (14-ounce / 397-g) can diced tomatoes, drained

½ cup sun-dried tomatoes

1 tablespoon dried oregano

1 teaspoon Italian seasoning

1 fresh jalapeño chile, stemmed, seeded, and minced

1 teaspoon salt

8 ounces (227 g) dried spaghetti, halved

1 cup spinach

Direction

1. Warm oil onSauté. Add onion and garlic and cook for 2 minutes until softened. Stir in pork and cook for 5 minutes. Stir in jalapeño, water, sun- dried tomatoes, Italian seasoning, oregano, diced tomatoes, and salt with the chicken; mix spaghetti and press to submerge into the sauce.
2. Seal the lid and cook on High Pressure for 9 minutes. Release the pressure quickly. Stir in spinach, close lid again, and simmer on Keep Warm for 5 minutes until spinach is wilted.

Per Serving

Calories: 621 | fat: 32.2g | protein: 29.1g | carbs: 53.9g | fiber: 5.9g | sodium: 738mg

Gouda Beef and Spinach Fettuccine

Prep time:

10 minutes | Cook time: 15 minutes | Serves 6

Ingredients

10 ounces (283 g) ground beef

1 pound (454 g) fettuccine pasta

1 cup gouda cheese, shredded

1 cup fresh spinach, torn

1 medium onion, chopped

2 cups tomatoes, diced

1 tablespoon olive oil

1 teaspoon salt

½ teaspoon ground black pepper

Direction

1. Heat the olive oil on Sauté mode in the Instant Pot. Stir-fry the beef and onion for 5 minutes. Add the pasta. Pour water enough to cover and season with salt and pepper. Cook on High Pressure for 5 minutes.
2. Do a quick release. Press Sauté and stir in the tomato and spinach; cook for 5 minutes. Top with Gouda to serve.

Per Serving

Calories: 493 | fat: 17.7g | protein: 20.6g | carbs: 64.3g | fiber: 9.5g | sodium: 561mg

Rigatoni and Zucchini Minestrone

Prep time:

20 minutes | Cook time: 7 minutes | Serves 4

Ingredients

3 tablespoons olive oil

1 onion, diced

1 celery stalk, diced

1 large carrot, peeled and diced

14 ounces (397 g) canned chopped tomatoes

4 ounces (113 g) rigatoni

3 cups water

1 cup chopped zucchini

1 bay leaf

1 teaspoon mixed herbs

¼ teaspoon cayenne pepper

½ teaspoon salt

¼ cup shredded Pecorino Romano cheese

1 garlic clove, minced

⅓ cup olive oil-based pesto

Direction

1. Heat oil on Sauté and cook onion, celery, garlic, and carrot for 3 minutes, stirring occasionally until the vegetables are softened. Stir in rigatoni, tomatoes, water, zucchini, bay leaf, herbs, cayenne, and salt.
2. Seal the lid and cook on High for 4 minutes. Do a natural pressure release for 5 minutes. Adjust the taste of the soup with salt and black pepper, and remove the bay leaf.
3. Ladle the soup into serving bowls and drizzle the pesto over. Serve with the garlic toasts.

Per Serving

Calories: 278 | fat: 23.4g | protein: 6.7g | carbs: 12.2g | fiber: 3.5g | sodium: 793mg

Asparagus and Broccoli Primavera Farfalle

Prep time:

15 minutes | Cook time: 12 minutes | Serves 4

Ingredients

1 bunch asparagus, trimmed, cut into 1-inch pieces

2 cups broccoli florets

3 tablespoons olive oil

3 teaspoons salt

10 ounces (283 g) egg noodles

3 garlic cloves, minced

2½ cups vegetable stock

½ cup heavy cream

1 cup small tomatoes, halved

¼ cup chopped basil

½ cup grated Parmesan cheese

Direction

1. Pour 2 cups of water, add the noodles, 2 tablespoons of olive oil, garlic and salt. Place a trivet over the water. Combine asparagus, broccoli, remaining olive oil and salt in a bowl. Place the vegetables on the trivet.
2. Seal the lid and cook on Steam for 12 minutes on High. Do a quick release. Remove the vegetables to a plate. Stir the heavy cream and tomatoes in the pasta. Press Sauté and simmer the cream until desired consistency. Gently mix in the asparagus and broccoli. Garnish with basil and Parmesan, to serve.

Per Serving

Calories: 544 | fat: 23.8g | protein: 18.5g | carbs: 66.1g | fiber: 6.0g | sodium: 2354mg

Super Cheesy Tagliatelle

Prep time:

10 minutes | Cook time: 20 minutes | Serves 6

Ingredients

¼ cup goat cheese, chevre

¼ cup grated Pecorino cheese

½ cup grated Parmesan

1 cup heavy cream

½ cup grated Gouda

2 tablespoons olive oil

1 tablespoon Italian Seasoning mix

1 cup vegetable broth

1 pound (454 g) tagliatelle

Direction

1. In a bowl, mix goat cheese, pecorino, Parmesan, and heavy cream. Stir in Italian seasoning. Transfer to your instant pot. Stir in the broth and olive oil.

2\. Seal the lid and cook on High Pressure for 4 minutes. Do a quick release.

1\. Meanwhile, drop the tagliatelle in boiling water and cook for 6 minutes.

2\. Remove the instant pot's lid and stir in the tagliatelle. Top with grated gouda and let simmer for about 10 minutes on Sauté mode.

Per Serving

Calories: 511 | fat: 22.0g | protein: 14.5g | carbs: 65.7g | fiber: 9.0g | sodium: 548mg

Chickpea Curry

Prep time:

10 minutes | Cook time: 24 minutes | Serves 4

Ingredients

½ cup raw chickpeas

1½ tablespoons cooking oil

½ cup chopped onions

1 bay leaf

½ tablespoon grated garlic

¼ tablespoon grated ginger

¾ cup water

1 cup fresh tomato purée

½ green chili, finely chopped

¼ teaspoon turmeric

½ teaspoon coriander powder

1 teaspoon chili powder

1 cup chopped baby spinach

Salt, to taste

Boiled white rice, for serving

Direction

1. Add the oil and onions to the Instant Pot. Sauté for 5 minutes.
2. Stir in ginger, garlic paste, green chili and bay leaf. Cook for 1 minute, then add all the spices.
3. Add the chickpeas, tomato purée and the water to the pot.
4. Cover and secure the lid. Turn its pressure release handle to the sealing position.
5. Cook on the Manual function with High Pressure for 15 minutes.
6. After the beep, do a Natural release for 20 minutes.
7. Stir in spinach and cook for 3 minutes on the Sauté setting.
8. Serve hot with boiled white rice.

Per Serving

Calories: 176 | fat: 6.8g | protein: 6.7g | carbs: 24.1g | fiber: 5.1g | sodium: 185mg

Cumin Quinoa Pilaf

Prep time:

5 minutes | Cook time: 5 minutes | Serves 2

Ingredients

2 tablespoons extra virgin olive oil

2 cloves garlic, minced

3 cups water

2 cups quinoa, rinsed

2 teaspoons ground cumin

2 teaspoons turmeric

Salt, to taste

1 handful parsley, chopped

Direction

1. Press the Sauté button to heat your Instant Pot.
2. Once hot, add the oil and garlic to the pot, stir and cook for 1 minute.
3. Add water, quinoa, cumin, turmeric, and salt, stirring well.
4. Lock the lid. Select the Manual mode and set the cooking time for 1 minute at High Pressure.
5. When the timer beeps, perform a natural pressure release for 10 minutes, then release any remaining pressure. Carefully remove the lid.
6. Fluff the quinoa with a fork. Season with more salt, if needed.
7. Sprinkle the chopped parsley on top and serve.

Per Serving

Calories: 384 | fat: 12.3g | protein: 12.8g | carbs: 57.4g | fiber: 6.9g | sodium: 448mg

Mint Brown Rice

Prep time:

5 minutes | Cook time: 22 minutes | Serves 2

Ingredients

2 cloves garlic, minced

¼ cup chopped fresh mint, plus more for garnish

1 tablespoon chopped dried chives

1 cup short- or long-grain brown rice

1½ cups water or low-sodium vegetable broth

½ to 1 teaspoon sea salt

Direction

1. Place the garlic, mint, chives, rice, and water in the Instant Pot. Stir to combine.
2. Secure the lid. Select the Manual mode and set the cooking time for 22 minutes at High Pressure.
3. Once cooking is complete, do a natural pressure release for 10 minutes, then release any remaining pressure. Carefully open the lid.
4. Add salt to taste and serve garnished with more mint.

Per Serving

Calories: 514 | fat: 6.6g | protein: 20.7g | carbs: 80.4g | fiber: 3.3g | sodium: 786mg

Rice and Sweet Potato Pilaf

Prep time:

15 minutes | Cook time: 10 minutes | Serves 4 to 6

Ingredients

2 tablespoons extra-virgin olive oil

1 onion, chopped fine

½ teaspoon table salt

2 garlic cloves, minced

1½ teaspoons ground turmeric

1 teaspoon ground coriander

⅛ teaspoon cayenne pepper

2 cups chicken broth

1½ cups long-grain white rice, rinsed

12 ounces (340 g) sweet potato, peeled, quartered lengthwise, and sliced ½ inch thick

½ preserved lemon, pulp and white pith removed, rind rinsed and minced (2 tablespoons)

½ cup shelled pistachios, toasted and chopped

¼ cup fresh cilantro leaves

¼ cup pomegranate seeds

Direction

1. Using highest Sauté function, heat oil in Instant Pot until shimmering. Add onion and salt and cook until onion is softened, about 5 minutes. Stir in garlic, turmeric, coriander, and cayenne and cook until fragrant, about 30 seconds. Stir in broth, rice, and sweet potato.
2. Lock lid in place and close pressure release valve. Select Manual function and cook for 4 minutes. Turn off Instant Pot and quick release pressure. Carefully remove lid, allowing steam to escape away from you.
3. Add preserved lemon and gently fluff rice with fork to combine. Lay clean dish towel over pot, replace lid, and let sit for 5 minutes. Season with salt and pepper to taste. Transfer to serving dish and sprinkle with pistachios, cilantro, and pomegranate seeds. Serve.

Per Serving

Calories: 698 | fat: 22.8g | protein: 36.8g | carbs: 85.5g | fiber: 5.9g | sodium: 802mg

Shrimp and Asparagus Risotto

Prep time:

15 minutes | Cook time: 58 minutes | Serves 4

Ingredients

1 tablespoon olive oil

1 pound (454 g) asparagus, trimmed and roughly chopped

1 cup spinach, chopped

1½ cups mushrooms, chopped

1 cup rice, rinsed and drained

1¼ cups chicken broth

¾ cup milk

1 tablespoon coconut oil

16 shrimp, cleaned and deveined

Salt and ground black pepper, to taste

¾ cup Parmesan cheese, shredded

Direction

1. Warm the oil on Sauté. Add spinach, mushrooms and asparagus and Sauté for 10 minutes until cooked through. Press Cancel. Add rice, milk and chicken broth to the pot as you stir.
2. Seal the lid, press Multigrain and cook for 40 minutes on High Pressure. Do a quick release, open the lid and put the rice on a serving plate.
3. Take back the empty pot to the pressure cooker, add coconut oil and press Sauté. Add shrimp and cook each side for 4 minutes until cooked through and turns pink. Set shrimp over rice, add pepper and salt for seasoning. Serve topped with shredded Parmesan cheese.

Per Serving

Calories: 385 | fat: 14.3g | protein: 16.5g | carbs: 48.4g | fiber: 4.1g | sodium: 771mg

Pancetta with Garbanzo Beans

Prep time:

10 minutes | Cook time: 38 minutes | Serves 6

Ingredients

3 strips pancetta

1 onion, diced

15 ounces (425 g) canned garbanzo beans

2 cups water

1 cup apple cider

2 garlic cloves, minced

½ cup ketchup

¼ cup sugar

1 teaspoon ground mustard powder

1 teaspoon salt

1 teaspoon black pepper

Fresh parsley, for garnish

Direction

1. Cook pancetta for 5 minutes, until crispy, on Sauté mode. Add onion and garlic, and cook for 3 minutes until soft. Mix in garbanzo beans, ketchup, sugar, salt, apple cider, mustard powder, water, and pepper.
2. Seal the lid, press Bean/Chili and cook on High Pressure for 30 minutes. Release pressure naturally for 10 minutes. Serve in bowls garnished with parsley.

Per Serving

Calories: 163 | fat: 5.7g | protein: 5.4g | carbs: 22.1g | fiber: 3.7g | sodium: 705mg

Brown Rice Stuffed Portobello Mushrooms

Prep time:

15 minutes | Cook time: 10 minutes | Serves 4

Ingredients

4 large portobello mushrooms, stems and gills removed

2 tablespoons olive oil

½ cup brown rice, cooked

1 tomato, seed removed and chopped

¼ cup black olives, pitted and chopped

1 green bell pepper, seeded and diced

½ cup feta cheese, crumbled

Juice of 1 lemon

½ teaspoon salt

½ teaspoon ground black pepper

Minced fresh cilantro, for garnish

1 cup vegetable broth

Direction

1. Brush the mushrooms with olive oil. Arrange the mushrooms in a single layer in an oiled baking pan. In a bowl, mix the rice, tomato, olives, bell pepper, feta cheese, lemon juice, salt, and black pepper.
2. Spoon the rice mixture into the mushrooms. Pour in the broth, seal the lid and cook on High Pressure for 10 minutes. Do a quick release. Garnish with fresh cilantro and serve immediately.

Per Serving

Calories: 190 | fat: 12.5g | protein: 5.9g | carbs: 15.2g | fiber: 2.6g | sodium: 682mg

Spinach and Ricotta Stuffed Pasta Shells

Prep time:

15 minutes | Cook time: 35 minutes | Serves 6

Ingredients

2 cups onion, chopped

1 cup carrot, chopped

3 garlic cloves, minced

3½ tablespoons olive oil,

1 (28-ounce / 794-g) canned tomatoes, crushed

12 ounces (340 g) conchiglie pasta

1 tablespoon olive oil

2 cups ricotta cheese, crumbled

1½ cups feta cheese, crumbled

2 cups spinach, chopped

¾ cup grated Pecorino Romano cheese

2 tablespoons chopped fresh chives

1 tablespoon chopped fresh dill

Salt and ground black pepper to taste

1 cup shredded Cheddar cheese

Direction

1. Warm olive oil on Sauté. Add onion, carrot, and garlic, and cook for 5 minutes until tender. Stir in tomatoes and cook for another 10 minutes. Remove to a bowl and set aside.
2. Wipe the pot with a damp cloth, add pasta and cover with enough water. Seal the lid and cook for 5 minutes on High Pressure. Do a quick release and drain the pasta. Lightly Grease olive oil to a baking sheet.
3. In a bowl, combine feta and ricotta cheese. Add spinach, Pecorino Romano cheese, dill, and chives, and stir well. Adjust the seasonings. Using a spoon, fill the shells with the mixture.
4. Spread 4 cups tomato sauce on the baking sheet. Place the stuffed shells over with seam-sides down and sprinkle Cheddar cheese atop. Use aluminum foil to the cover the baking dish.
5. Pour 1 cup of water in the pot of the Pressure cooker and insert the trivet. Lower the baking dish onto the trivet. Seal the lid, and cook for 15 minutes on High Pressure. Do a quick pressure release. Take away the foil. Place the stuffed shells to serving plates and top with tomato sauce before serving.

Per Serving

Calories: 730 | fat: 41.5g | protein: 30.0g | carbs: 62.7g | fiber: 10.6g | sodium: 966mg

Chili Halloumi Cheese with Rice

Prep time:

10 minutes | Cook time: 8 minutes | Serves 6

Ingredients

2 cups water

2 tablespoons brown sugar

2 tablespoons rice vinegar

1 tablespoon sweet chili sauce

1 tablespoon olive oil

1 teaspoon fresh minced garlic

20 ounces (567 g) Halloumi cheese, cubed

1 cup rice

¼ cup chopped fresh chives, for garnish

Direction

1. Heat the oil on Sauté and fry the halloumi for 5 minutes until golden brown. Set aside.
2. To the pot, add water, garlic, olive oil, vinegar, sugar, soy sauce, and chili sauce and mix well until smooth. Stir in rice noodles. Seal the lid and cook on High Pressure for 3 minutes. Release the pressure quickly. Split the rice between bowls. Top with fried halloumi and sprinkle with fresh chives before serving.

Per Serving

Calories: 534 | fat: 34.3g | protein: 24.9g | carbs: 30.1g | fiber: 1.0g | sodium: 652mg

Alphabetical Index

T

CPSIA information can be obtained
at www.ICGtesting.com
Printed in the USA
LVHW080134230521
688252LV00012B/507

9 781802 837735